Margaret Fawcett RGN RM LLSA is a trained general nurse, midwife and aromatherapist. She has worked as a midwife in locations as far apart as Saudi Arabia and London, where she spent time at The Garden Hospital, famous for its specialization in active birth techniques. She trained as an aromatherapist at the London School of Aromatherapy and has since combined her skills to work as an aromatherapist and midwife, currently based in Brighton, England.

D0168101

Aromatherapy for Pregnancy and Childbirth

MARGARET FAWCETT
RGN, RM, LLSA

E L E M E N T
Shaftesbury, Dorset • Boston, Massachusetts
Melbourne, Victoria

© Element Books Limited 1993
Text © Margaret Fawcett 1993

First published in the UK in 1993 by
Element Books Limited
Shaftesbury, Dorset SP7 8BP

Published in the USA in 1993 by
Element Books, Inc.
160 North Washington Street, Boston, MA 02114

Published in Australia in 1993 by
Element Books and distributed by
Penguin Australia Ltd
487 Maroondah Highway,
Ringwood, Victoria 3134

Reprinted 1994
Reprinted 1995
Reprinted 1996
Reprinted 1997
Reprinted 1998

All rights reserved.
No part of this book may be reproduced or utilized,
in any form or by any means, electronic or mechanical,
without prior permission in writing from the Publisher.

Designed by Roger Lightfoot
Artwork by David Gifford
Typeset by The Electronic Book Factory, Fife, Scotland
Printed and bound in the USA by Edwards Bros, Inc.

British Library Cataloguing in Publication
data available

Library of Congress Cataloging in Publication Data
Fawcett, Margaret.
Aromatherapy for pregnancy and childbirth Margaret Fawcett.
Includes bibliographical references and index.
1. Prenatal care. 2. Aromatherapy. 3. Pregnancy.
4. Childbirth. 5. Postnatal care. I. Title.
RG525.F38   1993   92–44943
618.2'4–dc20   CIP

ISBN 1–85230–390–5

TO MAM AND DAD

ACKNOWLEDGEMENTS

I should like to take this opportunity to thank the following for their advice and support during the writing of this book:

Helen Curtis, Maggie Craycroft, Karen Davison, Di Melck, Jacqui Hand, Ruth Holland (Midwifery Tutor, Royal Sussex County Hospital), Juliette Guernier, Georges O'Neil, Pat Scott, Ray Sherwin at Hermitage Oils, Margaret Wallace, and all the nurses on the Trevor Mann Baby Unit involved in the baby massage programme.

CONTENTS

AUTHOR'S NOTE

For the purposes of describing each stage of pregnancy I have used the following terms:

Very early pregnancy is approximately up to 8 weeks; early pregnancy from 8 up to 28 weeks; the middle weeks of pregnancy are from 28 to 36 weeks; and late pregnancy is from 37 weeks onwards.

These stages are approximate and if you are in any doubt please contact your midwife or aromatherapist before using any aromatherapy treatments to ensure that they are appropriate for that particular stage of your pregnancy.

INTRODUCTION

For many years I regularly purchased supplies of numerous essential oils, and used them occasionally around my home as room fragrances or in body preparations, but I was really unaware of their true healing powers – perhaps like many of you reading this now!

It was not until I began to work as a midwife in a hospital specializing in active birth that I began to develop a greater interest in aromatherapy. The lack of routine medication and technology gave me a clear insight into the natural birth processes and how readily nature responds to natural therapies, particularly aromatherapy. For not only do essential oils possess specific physical properties, but they also favourably influence the emotions by calming, stimulating and reassuring.

Impressed and eager to discover more about essential oils I began to study aromatherapy informally, then formally, at the London School of Aromatherapy. Eventually I established my own aromatherapy general practice specializing in treatments for pregnancy and childbirth, and baby massage.

In writing this book I have drawn mainly on my own experiences of using and prescribing aromatherapy for pregnancy and childbirth in my work both as a hospital-based and an independent midwife promoting homebirth, and as a professional aromatherapist. I have also used feedback from other midwives who regularly use essential oils in their own practices.

This book is not intended to replace the skills of a highly trained aromatherapist and midwife, but it will help you begin effective treatments immediately without waiting until you are able to acquire further professional advice.

Aromatherapy is only one of a great number of complementary treatments available for you to use during pregnancy and childbirth; but for the purposes of this book I have concentrated solely on the use of essential oils. If you are interested in other therapies, there are many excellent publications which focus on specific practices. At the end of this book you will find a list of useful addresses, including organizations that will supply further information and lists of suitably qualified therapists working in your area.

WHAT IS AROMATHERAPY?

Aromatherapy is a treatment using pure aromatic plant oils to enhance or restore well-being by stimulating the body's own natural healing processes.

These pure aromatic oils are usually known as essential oils. However, the word 'essential' is often misused in English to imply importance. True, these essential oils are important, for without them we would not be able to practise aromatherapy, but other languages are more specific. I have been told that Arabic for instance uses the word *ruh* which means 'spirit' or 'breath', implying that the essence is the very *life* of the plant from which it was obtained. This would perhaps go some way to explaining why aromatherapy is so effective, essential oils possessing the energy of air, earth, sun and water necessary for all plant life.

A BRIEF HISTORY OF AROMATHERAPY

Although the term 'aromatherapy' is fairly recent, the origins of the use of essential oils can be traced to ancient ceremonies. Perhaps the most well known are those of the ancient Egyptians who used plant extracts in ointments, pastes and incense, in cosmetics for beautifying, in medicines to treat the common illnesses of the day, and in religious practices, especially those surrounding birth and death.

This art of healing developed as knowledge spread from one civilization to another. The Greeks discovered various properties of plants and flowers for medicinal application, while the Arab world refined the method of extracting essential oils from plant material by distillation. In China and India the use of plant substances was widespread, as knowledge and experience passed from generation to generation.

Many of these practices are still in common use today, despite the destruction of many traditionally gathered plants by the intensive use of chemical pesticides.

Nearer home, a form of aromatherapy evolved using plants and flowers available in a less temperate climate, with more exotic vegetation introduced by returning explorers. These essential oils became invaluable in times of virulent infection, helping to protect the users from potentially fatal diseases, especially in the time of the great plagues.

Unfortunately, like many natural therapies, the use of plant extracts became less popular as chemical compounds were discovered and synthetic products, instead of traditional remedies, were prescribed by medical practitioners.

It was not until the 1920s that the term 'aromatherapy' was first introduced by the French scientist, Gattefossé. Having experienced the remarkable healing effects of essential oils after receiving treatment with lavender oil for burns sustained in a laboratory experiment, Gattefossé pioneered the renewed use of essential oils, publishing his book *Aromathérapie* in 1928.

Following Gattefossé came Dr Jean Valnet who applied his knowledge of essential oils in two very different ways. Working as a French army surgeon, Dr Valnet used essential oils to treat battle wounds, and later in his career used plant extracts to help rehabilitate patients with psychiatric disorders.

At around the same time another French national, Madame Marguerite Maury, a biochemist, developed special massage techniques while using essential oils in therapeutic as well as cosmetic applications.

Today, scientific research continues, and essential oils have become readily available for use in everyday life as aromatherapy increases in popularity.

Although the application of aromatherapy during pregnancy and childbirth is fairly recent, a rapidly growing number of both mothers and professionals are using essential oils. Many midwives are now training in aromatherapy, and aromatherapists and the use of essential oils are welcomed in all maternity hospitals. Aromatherapy is now valued as part of a wide range of therapies available as a treatment for most conditions that may develop during pregnancy, as a non-invasive aid to natural birth, and for promoting rapid recovery, as well as being an effective supplement to any necessary medical or technological treatments.

HOW AROMATHERAPY WORKS

Described chemically, essential oils have a simple structure which makes them easily absorbed by the body; yet they are complex in that they are made up of many active constituents. This gives an essential oil its unique aroma, and also explains why one essential oil may have several therapeutic qualities. This combination is much more effective than using a single isolated compound which is what most chemists attempt to separate from organic material for use in synthetic preparations.

Wherever essential oils are used, the aroma is detected by fine hairs in the nose. This produces nerve impulses which pass through nerve cells to a part of the brain known as the lymbic system. The lymbic system controls memory and emotion, and is also closely connected with the pituitary gland which governs hormonal function.

Essential oils are also easily absorbed through the skin and in a small part through the lungs. They are then carried around the body by the circulation. So either by way of detection or absorption, essential oils can very quickly affect all systems of the body.

Some essential oils work directly on the circulation or on specific organs of the body; some regulate the metabolism by sedating or stimulating; others by association. In the same way that a certain perfume can remind you of a friend or lover (or if, like me, the zest of tangerines always reminds you Christmas), so specific essential oils work by association with positive emotions or pleasant memories of events you have previously experienced.

Because the essential oils that we use in aromatherapy are pure plant products, they do not produce side-effects and are non-addictive, unlike many of today's conventional medicines. When the correct essential oils are selected aromatherapy works quickly and effectively. Regular treatments with essential oils will help you maintain optimum health and vitality as well as directly treating the specific problems that may develop during pregnancy and childbirth, and will also supplement most other therapies whether complementary or orthodox.

ENCOURAGING HEALTHY ATTITUDES TOWARDS PREGNANCY

Pregnancy is not an illness, but it is important that during your pregnancy you develop a holistic approach to your health in that you regularly assess your physical, emotional and spiritual needs.

Eating a nourishing diet and having adequate amounts of rest and exercise are vital to maintaining your own well-being, as well as that of your baby who is dependent on you to provide all the requirements for growth and development. Almost every substance you choose to put into or on to your body, such as essential oils, minerals and vitamins, as well as toxic chemicals, alcohol and tobacco, all have an effect. But remember your baby does not have the opportunity to reject what is harmful.

If illness does develop, try to identify the underlying cause rather than being content simply to treat the symptoms. We all occasionally take stimulants such as tea or coffee when we are feeling tired and really need to rest, or take painkillers for headaches when we should try to eliminate the cause by reducing stress and tension or environmental pollutants such as poor artificial lighting or faulty air-conditioning. Trying to discover the source of a problem will help you work towards preventing a recurrence of similar conditions. But what is particularly important during pregnancy is that this method of diagnosis and treatment will help you recognize the natural signals coming from within your body warning that more serious illness may be developing.

You will discover that pregnancy is a time of great emotional change. At times we all experience conflicting emotions, and unfortunately the months of pregnancy will not protect you from these feelings, and can actually make you more vulnerable and increase your apprehensions.

At some point, usually in the early weeks, you may, like many women, feel frightened or resentful of the effects that pregnancy is having on your life and relationships with your partner, family and friends. In the later weeks you may become almost terrified at the thought of giving birth, or failing to give birth normally, or that your baby will be affected by some disability. These feelings are normal. But open discussion of these negative thoughts will prevent very real anxieties from becoming exaggerated or adversely affecting your overall attitude towards yourself, your baby or your supporters.

Using aromatherapy will help you treat yourself as a whole person by stimulating and strengthening a positive balance and a harmony of mind, body and spirit. The testing time of pregnancy and childbirth will help you develop a tremendous feeling of inner strength and resourcefulness previously undiscovered.

2

INSTRUCTIONS
FOR USING
ESSENTIAL OILS

PREPARING AND USING ESSENTIAL OILS

Preparing and using essential oils is not difficult as long as you follow a few basic rules. Remember to wash your hands before and after handling essential oils. Do not let essential oils come into contact with your eyes. If this does happen rinse immediately with clear water and, if necessary, seek further medical advice.

Choose a time to prepare your essential oils when you will not be interrupted, especially when you are adding essential oils to carrier oils as it is important that you count the drops accurately as too strong a mixture can cause skin irritation, while a weak solution will not have the desired effect. 'Carrier oils' are vegetable oils used to dilute essential oils prior to massage or topical treatments (see Chapters 3 and 7).

Always mix your essential oils in an area away from food or substances with strong-smelling odours as these will not only contaminate the essential oils, but can also affect the subtle process of blending, when an accurate sense of smell is required.

Work on a firm surface that can be easily cleaned, as essential oils and carrier oils can damage certain surfaces. Have a roll of kitchen towel handy to mop up spills and wipe clean bottles. Some essential oils have a tendency towards spontaneous combustion. Although this is very rare, put wipes immediately into an outside bin.

Before you start, make sure that all your equipment is clean and dried well. Plastic kitchen spoons can be used for measuring carrier oils, and you can use a funnel to transfer carrier oils from large containers to small bottles. These items can be easily obtained from chemists or kitchen supply shops.

Essential oils, although expensive to purchase initially, do go a long way. When you buy 10mls of pure essential oil you will get approximately 200 drops of essential oil from each bottle.

When using essential oils during pregnancy and child-birth the dilution should always be 2 per cent: therefore add 2 drops of essential oil to every 5mls (1 teaspoon) of carrier oil. About 30mls of carrier oil is sufficient for a full body massage. So, for example, add 12 drops of essential oil to 30mls of carrier oil. This rule applies whether you are using one essential oil or a combination of several.

Your essential oils, carrier oils and mixed preparations should always be stored away from direct sunlight where they cannot be affected by extremes of temperature or humidity, and like other medicines should always be kept out of the reach of children and animals.

AROMATIC BATHS

When adding essential oils to your bath water do not use more than a total of 6 drops. Sprinkle the essential oil on to the surface of still water. Then mix well before entering, although essential oils will not dissolve in water, but will float on the surface when the water settles. For a more uniform solution and to prevent the essential oil sticking to the sides of the bath, you may wish to mix your essential oils in a little cow's milk or sweet almond oil before adding to the water. Your bath should be comfortably warm, but not hot. Hot water will cause most essential oils to evaporate before your skin has had time to absorb them.

Soak for approximately 10–15 minutes. Do not use soap as this affects the chemical composition of all essential oils destroying both their aroma and healing qualities.

COMPRESSES

Fill a basin with hot or cold water as required. Sprinkle 6 drops of essential oil on to the surface of the water. Do not mix. Use a clean suitably sized piece of material (eg, flannel for your breast, small towel for your back) and dip the material into the water so that it picks up as much of the essential oil as possible. Wring out the excess water and apply the compress to the affected area. Cover your compress with a piece of waterproof material to help retain the desired temperature. Replace your compress as soon as it reaches body temperature.

FOOTBATHS

Fill a bowl or basin with tepid water, then add a total of 4 drops of essential oil. Mix well. Then soak your feet for 10–15 minutes. Do not use soap (see *Aromatic Baths* above).

INTERNAL MEDICATION

In my opinion *no* essential oils should be taken internally. This practice is unnecessary, and potentially extremely dangerous. The oils are effectively absorbed by external application; if the desired result is not achieved they can easily be removed with a mild soap and water solution to prevent any more of the essence from entering your circulation. Once swallowed essential oils cannot be easily neutralized.

As well as tasting unpleasant, essential oils are known irritants to the stomach lining. Therefore if taken internally over a long period of time they will certainly cause damage to delicate tissues.

LOCAL WASHES

This mixture can be used as a final rinse after washing. Add a total of 4 drops of essential oil to 1 litre of warm water (an empty mineral water bottle can be kept specially for this purpose). Use the entire contents each time, preparing fresh mixture when required.

SITZ-BATHS AND BIDETS

Fill a bath or bidet with warm water to reach hip level. If a bath or bidet is not available, keep a washing-up bowl especially for this purpose. Sprinkle a total of 4 drops of essential oil on to the surface of the water, then mix well before soaking.

MASSAGE OILS

Your massage oil should consist of 2 per cent essential oil to 98 per cent carrier oil. For example: 2 drops of essential oil should be added for every 5mls (1 teaspoon) of carrier oil.

When prepared, the mixture – if kept in an airtight

container – should last for several weeks, but I prefer to prepare a fresh mixture just before giving a massage, mixing the essential oils in a shallow dish or saucer so that I can easily dip my hands into the oil without breaking the rhythm of my massage strokes.

Do not massage if there is:

• A rise in body temperature
• Broken or infected skin
• Recent scars
• Fractures or dislocations
• Swollen, hot or painful joints
• Varicose veins

VAPORIZATION

Ceramic essential oil vaporizers are available from most health shops or suppliers of essential oils, and come in many different shapes and sizes. All work in the same way, by warming the oil and water mixture causing the solution to evaporate.

Fill the top bowl with water and then add a total of 4–10 drops of essential oil, depending on the size of the vaporizer. Insert a lighted candle underneath the bowl. This warms the water and oil which then evaporate together.

Alternatively, simply add essential oils to a bowl of just boiled water, and the essential oils will evaporate with the steam.

CAUTIONS

When using citrus oils, especially Lemon oil, you must take special care. These essential oils have very concentrated astringent qualities and can irritate your skin. When preparing your massage blends add only half the prescribed number of drops of citrus oils that is, 1 drop of essential oil to every 5mls of carrier oil, and just 3 drops to your bath water. If you feel that your skin is particularly sensitive reduce the dose further by adding 1 drop of essential oil to every 10mls of carrier oil, and use only 2 drops in your bath water, or avoid using citrus oils altogether, and continue your treatments using a recommended alternative essential oil.

You must also avoid sunbathing for at least 4 hours after applying citrus oils to your skin, particularly Bergamot oil, as direct exposure to the sun can cause minor tissue burns and a permanent discoloration of the skin.

If you are using the same type of essential oil over a long period of time, allow a break of 7 continuous days at the end of every 3 weeks. This will prevent an accumulation of essential oils in your body tissues. During this time you can continue your treatments by using another essential oil with similar healing properties. This way you can continue to use the same essential oil for as long as you wish, for unlike modern chemical treatments, such as antibiotic therapy, you will not develop immunity. Each treatment will be as effective as the first, even if you use the same essential oil over a period of days, weeks or even months.

3

THE MAIN ESSENTIAL OILS USED DURING PREGNANCY AND CHILDBIRTH

METHODS OF EXTRACTION

Essential oils are extracted from flowers, fruit, herbs and trees in many regions around the world, each essential oil having unique characteristics, colour and fragrance. (This is true even of essential oils that have been obtained from plants of the same species but grown in different areas.) Essential oils are not greasy, but have a consistency which is rather like alcohol.

The most common method of extraction is by distillation. The plant material is immersed in boiling water or steam, which causes the essence to be released in vapour. This is gathered and then cooled, and the essential oil is collected as it separates from the water.

Most citrus oils are obtained by direct pressure. The peel of the fruit is squeezed and the aromatic oil gathered from the juice.

Another method uses a solvent which absorbs the essence as it flows through tanks containing plant material. The liquid is then distilled to obtain a semi-solid perfume.

Enfleurage is a method used to capture the fragrance of delicate flowers such as Rose or Jasmine. It is the most time-consuming and expensive method, which you will find is reflected in the price of these essential oils.

This process involves using frames coated with lard on to which flower petals are pressed. When the lard is eventually saturated with aromatic constituents, a process that can take several days, it is cleaned with alcohol to wash out the oil it has absorbed. The alcohol is then evaporated off.

THE ESSENTIAL OILS AND THEIR RELEVANT PROPERTIES

The following essential oils have been selected for their known effectiveness in treating specific conditions that may develop during pregnancy and childbirth, as well as helping reduce tension and aid relaxation. Each essential oil has powerful physically healing qualities, as well as a more subtle effect on the emotions.

Beside each essential oil you will find its botanical name. This is important for it can avoid confusion when ordering essential oils from your supplier. This is followed by a brief description of the relevant properties of each essential oil for use during pregnancy and childbirth.

Bergamot (Citrus bergamia)

Expressed from the rind of an orange-like fruit native to Italy, Bergamot has a refreshing citrus aroma. It is effective in helping treat the irritation, stinging and tenderness caused by urinary tract infections which may develop during pregnancy. Bergamot has uplifting qualities, helping relieve depression and anxiety. Safe throughout pregnancy. *Caution*: phototoxic.

Chamomile, Roman (Anthemis nobilis)

Distilled from flowers common in Europe, Chamomile has a sweet fragrance and possesses analgesic and anti-inflammatory properties effective for relieving muscle spasm experienced as backache, or discomfort due to infection within the urinary tract. It is a good conditioner for fair hair. This essential oil is gentle and calming to the emotions. Safe after 16 weeks.

Clary Sage (Salvia sclarea)

The oil is distilled from the whole plant, which is a herb with a nutty fragrance found in the Mediterranean region. Clary Sage helps tone and stimulate the uterus and can be applied to induce labour or strengthen contractions during childbirth. It also works well as a sedative for stress and tension. Use only in late pregnancy to induce labour and during childbirth. *Caution*: do not use while drinking alcohol.

Cypress (Cupressus sempervirens)

Distilled from the cones and twigs of the Cypress tree found in the Mediterranean region, this is a powerful astringent and circulatory tonic that is useful as a treatment for varicose veins and haemorrhoids. Cypress also helps relieve excessive foot perspiration commonly experienced during pregnancy. Safe throughout pregnancy.

Frankincense (Boswellia thurifera)

Distilled from the resin exuding from the bark of a tree native to Arabia and East Africa, this oil has a unique fragrance. Frankincense has a toning effect on the skin and helps clear the lungs. This penetrating essential oil is effective in helping the user cope with extremely stressful situations, inducing a state of concentration. Safe throughout pregnancy.

Geranium (Pelargonium graveolens)

Geranium oil is distilled from the leaves, stalks and flowers of the plant, which is native to South Africa. It has a sweet, rose fragrance and is good for poor circulation, oedema, breast engorgement, stress and anxiety. It helps to restore hormonal equilibrium. Safe throughout pregnancy.

Jasmine (Jasminum grandiflorum)

This essential oil is obtained from the flowers of a plant native to the East. Jasmine, which has a sweet aroma, will help restore hormone balance following childbirth, and is also calming and relaxing, encouraging optimism and confidence. Safe after 16 weeks.

Lavender (Lavandula angustifolia)

Distilled from the flower, Lavender has a wide range of therapeutic qualities:

- Analgesic
- Encourages the healing of damaged tissue
- Prevents excess scar tissue developing
- Relieves headaches
- Settles the stomach
- Stimulates the immune system, helping protect the user from infection
- Useful in helping treat constipation
- Has a soothing and gentle presence for helping reduce high blood pressure

Lavender can also be frequently used to enhance the action of many other essential oils. Safe throughout pregnancy.

Lemon (Citrus limonum)

Expressed from the peel of the fruit of the Lemon tree which originates in the East, this essential oil has a clear fresh fragrance. It helps tone the circulation and reduce tissue congestion. Lemon also stimulates the immune system, improving the user's resistance to infection. Safe throughout pregnancy. *Caution*: phototoxic, may cause irritation.

Mandarin (Citrus madurensis)

Expressed from the peel of the fruit of a tree native to the East, Mandarin has a sweet refreshing fragrance, which encourages optimism, and also helps soothe and settle the nervous system and digestive tract. A bright, gentle and calming essential oil. Safe throughout pregnancy. *Caution*: possibly phototoxic.

Neroli (Citrus aurantium)

Distilled from flowers native to the East, Neroli has a delicate floral fragrance. It acts as a sedative for the nervous system, relieving stress and states of depression. It is also good for nourishing the growing layer of the skin in treatments for stretch marks. Safe throughout pregnancy.

Orange (Citrus sirensis)

Expressed from the peel of the Orange; the tree originating in the East. With its tropical fragrance, Orange helps tone and stimulate the digestive tract, and is useful for digestive upsets. It is bright and energizing. Safe throughout pregnancy. *Caution*: phototoxic.

Patchouli (Pogostemon patchouli)

Distilled from the leaves of the plant, a herb native to Indonesia, Patchouli has a warm earthy aroma, good for treating inflamed skin and preventing the development of infection. It also works well as a nerve tonic and is useful in helping overcome anxiety. Safe throughout pregnancy.

Peppermint (Mentha piperita)

Distilled from the whole plant, a herb found throughout northern temperate regions, Peppermint is valuable for helping treat all digestive problems, nausea and headaches. It also relieves breast engorgement by reducing the circulation to breast tissue. It may be used in footbaths to refresh and deodorize tired and aching feet. It is stimulating and invigorating. Safe after 16 weeks. *Caution*: skin irritant in concentration.

Rose *(Rosa damascena)*

Derived from the flower petals and having an elegant fragrance, this oil is relaxing and soothing when experiencing anger or intense emotions. Rose also helps regulate hormone balance following childbirth. Safe after 16 weeks.

Rosemary *(Rosmarinus officinalis)*

Distilled from the whole plant, which is native to the Mediterranean, this is a warming oil good for encouraging the circulation needed for the production and flow of breast milk. It is also a good conditioner for dark hair, and is useful for states of tiredness and fatigue. Safe in late pregnancy only. *Caution*: avoid in cases of high blood pressure.

Sandalwood *(Santalum album)*

Distilled from the heartwood of the tree native to India, Sandalwood has a sweet exotic fragrance, and is a powerful antiseptic, useful when treating urinary tract infections. It is relaxing and supportive. Safe throughout pregnancy.

Ti-Tree *(Melaleuca alternifolia)*

Distilled from the leaves of trees native to Australia, Ti-Tree has antibacterial, antifungal and antiviral properties which aid the healing of damaged tissue while helping prevent the development of infection. Safe throughout pregnancy.

Ylang Ylang (Cananga odorata)

Ylang ylang oil is distilled from the freshly-picked flowers of a tree native to tropical Asia. It has a sweet, floral, slightly spicy scent. Ylang ylang is good for high blood pressure, stress and anxiety. It is an anti-depressant. Safe throughout pregnancy.

CHOOSING AN ESSENTIAL OIL

If this is your first experience of using aromatherapy you may, like many women, have some difficulty in deciding which essential oil will be the most effective in treating a particular disorder, in that there may be a choice of several essential oils to treat one specific condition, as properties of some oils overlap. When faced with a choice, if possible try to inhale a little of the vapour of each essential oil, and then select the one that you personally find favourable, because if it smells right then that essential oil will be the most effective for you. Similarly, if you find that a recommended essential oil smells unpleasant do try an alternative, because you will find that this essential oil will probably not work for you no matter how fabled its healing properties.

If you feel that you are still experiencing difficulty in choosing an essential oil that is just right for you, a visit to an aromatherapist may help. An aromatherapist, especially one who has experience of treating women during pregnancy and childbirth, will be more objective in their assessment of your condition, and will select essential oils that are right for you at that treatment session, as well as being able to suggest other essential oils for later use at home.

CARRIER OILS

Carrier, or base or fixed oils as they are sometimes known, are used to dilute essential oils prior to giving massage or topical treatments, essential oils being too concentrated to be applied directly to large areas of the body. Carrier oils also assist in the absorption of essential oils through the skin into the circulation.

You can use any type of vegetable oil as your carrier oil, but do not use mineral based oils as these are incompatible with essential oils and are not absorbed by the skin.

Sweet Almond Oil

This carrier oil should not be confused with Bitter Almond oil which is poisonous. There are many types of carrier oils available, but I personally use Sweet Almond oil for 99 per cent of treatments. Sweet Almond is fine, colourless and odourless, and is very easily absorbed by the skin. It contains Vitamin E which is useful in the treatment of skin conditions, as well as acting as a preservative which will extend the life of your massage preparations. You will find that other carrier oils will go rancid fairly quickly, and so for this reason when prepared with essential oils they should be used immediately.

Grapeseed Oil

This carrier oil is more economical than Sweet Almond oil and has a lighter texture.

Avocado Oil

This oil is rich and moisturizing, and is good as a treatment for dry or dehydrated skin.

Jojoba Oil

This is a fine and penetrating oil, good to use as a moisturizer for the face, or to add shine to dry or dull hair.

Wheatgerm Oil

Containing Vitamins A, B, C and E this carrier oil is particularly nourishing for growing skin and scar tissue, stimulating the production of skin cells. I would suggest that Wheatgerm oil is not a good carrier oil due to the wheaty smell and because it is too thick and sticky to apply smoothly. It can, however, be used added as a 5 per cent concentration to massage preparations, when it will also act as a preservative.

Evening Primrose Oil

The herb being called the King's Cure All, Evening Primrose oil is effective in the treatment of menstrual and nervous disorders, allergies and the topical treatment of skin conditions such as eczema and psoriasis. Evening Primrose oil is safe to take internally when specially prepared by the manufacturer, the dose being 8 drops twice a day for 10 days, then gradually reducing to a minimum of 4 drops twice a day. Many people experience immediate tonic effects after taking this oil internally. Unfortunately the effect is usually short lived, but does indicate that the person needed the supplement and it is likely to have beneficial effects in the long term.

However, many people find that this oil is rather unpleasant due to the wheaty taste as it contains 5 per cent wheatgerm which acts as a preservative. In this case you may find it more palatable when added to cold foods, or add a percentage to another carrier oil and use in topical applications.

Alternatively, Evening Primrose oil is available in capsule form. Follow the manufacturer's instructions as regards dosage.

ESSENTIAL OILS TO AVOID DURING PREGNANCY AND CHILDBIRTH

If used wisely essential oils carry no danger of harming you or your baby. However, aromatherapy is a very powerful treatment and should always be approached with caution.

During your pregnancy you will develop heightened sensitivity to all external influences, and essential oils are no exception. If any skin irritation, rash, redness or soreness develops, you should discontinue treatment and immediately wash your skin with soap and water to clear away any residue. You should also drink some extra water.

There are a number of essential oils that must be completely avoided during your pregnancy. These are described as toxic in that their effects could harm both you and your baby. There are others that should only be used in late pregnancy or during labour because their effects could stimulate contractions. And finally there are other essential oils that should only be used to aid your recovery following the birth of your baby.

Essential oils to be completely avoided during your pregnancy

- Aniseed
- Armoise
- Arnica (not to be confused with homoeopathic remedy)
- Basil
- Camphor

- Caraway
- Cinnamon
- Clove
- Cedarwood
- Fennel
- Hyssop
- Marjoram
- Mugwort
- Myrrh
- Nutmeg
- Origanum
- Pennyroyal
- Sage
- Savory
- Tansy
- Tarragon
- Thuja
- Thyme
- Wintergreen

Essential oils that must be used with caution during pregnancy

- Chamomile
- Clary Sage
- Peppermint
- Rose
- Rosemary

If you have a history of bleeding during your pregnancy or of miscarriage, or if you believe that you have a condition that may contra-indicate the use of essential oils, or even if you are unsure about the safety of certain essential oils, do seek further advice from your aromatherapist before you start treatments as they will be aware of up to date scientific research.

Like most therapies, aromatherapy should be avoided in the very early weeks of your pregnancy. This is a very important time of development during which your baby is extremely vulnerable to external influences. In the weeks following you can slowly begin to introduce the use of essential oils. Peppermint and Rosemary may be used in late pregnancy with caution, but are thought to be toxic in early pregnancy. Do not use Rosemary if you develop high blood pressure during your pregnancy or labour as it may unduly stimulate the circulation if high blood pressure develops.

You should only use Clary Sage, Rose, Jasmine or any other essential oil that works on the uterus or that influences hormone balance, during labour to stimulate contractions or after the birth of your baby to aid your recovery.

Following the birth of your baby, most essential oils are safe to use, but I would recommend that initially you use only those oils specifically recommended to aid your recovery.

Do not use essential oils in your baby massage preparations as these are much too powerful for small babies, and there is a danger that the essential oil may accidentally enter the eyes or be ingested as your baby sucks fingers or fists. Remember to remove all traces of essential oils prior to breast feeding – this can be done quite easily using a mild soap and water solution.

PLANNING FOR PREGNANCY AND CHILDBIRTH

Your pregnancy and the birth of your baby are major life experiences and as such you may wish to plan for these events well before you actually become pregnant.

This interval of planning will allow you time to concentrate on any aspects of your health or life style that are of particular concern to you – for example, the health and fitness of both yourself and your partner, with special attention to diet, rest and exercise.

You may also like to take this opportunity to become more familiar with aromatherapy and the use of essential oils, visiting an aromatherapist if you require.

It is also a good idea to begin to consider what other types of professional care you would like, and how and where you would prefer to give birth, as well as preparing emotionally for pregnancy and childbirth. This will help you adjust to your changing role as you become a parent, and consider the relationship between yourself, your partner, family and friends.

PRECONCEPTUAL CARE

If you are planning for pregnancy and childbirth you may initially decide to visit your local health centre for preconceptual care and advice before you become pregnant.

This visit will help you make sure that you are physically fit and well before you conceive, as well as providing an opportunity for you to discuss any apprehensions that you may have concerning pregnancy and childbirth.

At this appointment, the physical assessment is usually fairly thorough and includes a general examination of your circulation, heart, lungs and blood pressure. You will be asked to provide a urine specimen that can be tested to exclude the presence of any abnormalities, such as infections, and your weight will be measured.

This examination will be followed by a general discussion of any health problems that you may be experiencing, plus advice on diet and exercise should you require it. With your consent, the examination may also include a vaginal examination. This is necessary in order to check the health of your uterus, ovaries and cervix (the neck of your womb) by cervical smear.

You may be advised to stop or change your method of contraception as it is preferable that all internal (the coil) or hormonal methods of contraception are not used for at least three months prior to conception in order to allow your natural menstrual cycle to be re-established. The expected date of the birth of your baby can then be accurately calculated from the first day of your last menstrual period (when you begin to try to conceive remember to record this important date each month).

You may also be offered special blood tests to make sure that you are not anaemic (low in blood iron). If you are anaemic this can be corrected by including more iron rich foods in your diet, such as dried fruits, green leafy vegetables, pulses, seeds and grains, or if really necessary by taking iron supplements.

Your blood can also be examined to make sure that you are immune to Rubella (German Measles) which, if contracted during your pregnancy, can seriously impair the development of your baby. If you are susceptible to Rubella, you will be offered the vaccine and, once taken, you should avoid becoming pregnant for three months until immunity has safely become established.

You may also be asked about your own and your partner's family history, to detect any condition, such as high blood pressure or diabetes, which could possibly affect you during pregnancy, or which could affect the development of your baby. Details of other pregnancies are also important as their outcome can affect the care that you will receive. In other words, if you have already experienced difficult pregnancies or births you may require closer monitoring during pregnancy and the birth of your next baby.

Congenital disorders are rare in couples who are fit and well, but if you are particularly worried or have a family history of congenital disability, you may require special tests and counselling prior to pregnancy.

Pregnancy and childbirth are deeply emotional experiences. If you feel that you have or are suffering from emotional difficulties, anxieties or depression you may wish to consider special counselling. This can be continued throughout your pregnancy and after the birth of your baby to help you adjust to your changing role and to cope with the demands of parenthood.

Planning for pregnancy and childbirth will also give you time to consider other aspects of parenthood, such as the impact on your finances, loss of income should you have to stop working, and housing should you need a larger home.

This period of planning is also a good time for you to select an aromatherapist if you do not already have one (see *Appendix*). Try to select a therapist who will offer treatments and support during pregnancy and, if possible, childbirth if you are considering being attended by an aromatherapist during the birth of your baby.

You can also take time to become familiar with the essential oils themselves during this period if you have not previously used them. You will find that with practice they are very easy to prepare and use and you will soon come to recognize your own likes and dislikes.

During pregnancy and childbirth most women develop a heightened sensitivity, particularly to aromas, and you may find that you no longer like to use a certain essential oil that was perhaps your favourite before you became pregnant. This is often due to your own body selecting what is right for you to use at that time. Trust this instinct – even though the range of essential oils is restricted during pregnancy and childbirth there are still plenty to choose from. When treating a woman during pregnancy and childbirth I very often select a handful of essential oils that possess the relevant healing properties and leave the woman to decide which essential oil she prefers.

Remember that this preconceptual care is also available to the prospective father who should be encouraged to participate. You may also feel that you would like to have preconceptual counselling with your partner at a later date to discuss your anxieties together.

IMPROVING YOUR FERTILITY

Providing that you and your partner are physically fit and well, and have not previously suffered any illness that may have affected your reproductive system, you should not experience any problems with your fertility.

Having said this, however, there are a surprising number of couples who do have problems with their fertility for no apparent reason. It is possible that this may be the result of the long-term use of hormonal methods of contraception which has affected the natural menstrual cycle and which can make ovulation difficult to predict. If, in preparation for pregnancy, you have decided no longer to use these methods of contraception, aromatherapy may help you improve your fertility by helping restore your natural cycle.

Used as a belly or back massage Neroli, Rose and Jasmine will help influence the emotions to help establish a natural hormone balance, while Clary Sage has a cleansing and tonic action on the uterus. These essential oils should be used daily, either singly or in combination. Stop the treatments for the 7 days when your menstrual period should take place, and then resume treatments for the following three weeks. Follow the same routine until you are satisfied that your normal cycle is re-established. Then discontinue treatments once you intend to become pregnant.

Many other problems concerning fertility are often due to the effects of stress and tensions which unfortunately could be due in part to the actual planning of your pregnancy. If you or your partner are worried or anxious do try to discuss this apprehension openly together and seek further professional advice if necessary, for stress can manifest in many ways, and can affect fertility if left unchecked. You and your partner will both benefit from aromatic baths and massage. Again discontinue using aromatherapy treatments once you intend to conceive.

Use the specific essential oils previously described to help regulate your menstrual cycle, or choose your own favourites if you prefer. Men often prefer the less flowery tones of Sandalwood, Patchouli or Frankincense.

If you feel that you or your partner are affected by stress it may also be a good idea to visit your aromatherapist on a regular basis. As well as giving you the opportunity to discuss your apprehensions, these regular treatments will enhance the action of essential oils and help promote a more relaxed attitude towards pregnancy and childbirth.

REST AND EXERCISE

Ideally we would all have as much rest as we need, but unfortunately the pressure of our daily lives means that this is rarely the case. As physical fitness during pregnancy and childbirth will depend as much on the amount of rest you receive as on exercise it it important to try to establish a routine, resting whenever possible.

It is equally important to develop an exercise routine. I

am not suggesting that you suddenly begin serious physical training, but do try to do as much exercise as your body feels comfortable with.

Try to develop an exercise programme that suits you, concentrating on exercises that develop the muscles involved during pregnancy and childbirth, such as pelvic floor exercises. Your pelvic floor muscles (those muscles that you tighten to stop urinating midstream) are a very important group of muscles for, not only do they assist your bladder control and help support your growing uterus during pregnancy, but they also help guide your baby through your birth canal during the process of childbirth.

Other forms of exercise, such as yoga, walking and swimming, are gentle enough to be continued during pregnancy and will also help your recovery and keep you looking and feeling good.

It is advisable that you do not try to reduce your weight by dieting as this may lead to a loss of vital vitamins and minerals necessary for the initial development of your baby. You should, however, examine your diet and try to reduce an excess intake of sugar and carbohydrates, as well as considering the effects of alcohol, drugs and tobacco upon you and your baby.

THE TYPE OF CARE YOU WOULD LIKE

As well as becoming physically fit and well prior to pregnancy and childbirth, you may also like to take time to find a suitable aromatherapist and to plan whom you would like to provide your professional maternity care.

Some women opt for hospital care at their local maternity unit, especially if they have previously experienced problems with their fertility or other pregnancies, or if they require specialist care. Others choose to be cared for alternately by their own general practitioner and the maternity unit. This saves on travelling and waiting time.

You may prefer simply to visit your own general practitioner, particularly if you have a good relationship and wish to stay at that practice for your care following the birth of your baby. This type of care is usually shared with your community midwife, whom you can choose to consult for *all* of your maternity care if you so wish.

This type of care is preferred by many women, especially those who are planning to have their community midwife with them for the birth of their baby in hospital, or if they are planning a home birth. In both cases you will be attended by a midwife whom you will have had an opportunity to meet during your pregnancy, and who will continue to provide care for you and your baby at home in the days following the birth.

You may also be fortunate enough to have the option of employing an independent midwife (see *Useful Addresses*). Independent midwives are self employed, and charges vary tremendously. Usually the fees are agreed in advance between you and your midwife. All care during the antenatal, birth and postnatal period is provided in your own home, during which time a close relationship is able to form between you, your family and your midwife.

PLANNING FOR THE BIRTH

Part of planning for pregnancy and childbirth is beginning to think about where and how you would prefer to give birth.

You may think that this is planning much too far in advance, but this is the time when you can take a more objective view and be able to take into consideration all the options available and not leave this major decision to the last few weeks of your pregnancy when you may find yourself frantically looking for an environment that suits you.

Start by becoming well informed. Talk to your midwife, general practitioner and local birth support groups to see what is on offer, and to other mothers who have had birth experiences similar to the one that you would prefer.

It may help you to list your preferences which can later be constructed into a birth plan, considering options such as the use of aromatherapy, drugs and monitoring during childbirth, as well as how you would prefer to give birth – such as squatting, or water birth. Your midwife will be able to advise you if you need assistance or information, particularly regarding your local Health Authority policies.

Many women decide to have a hospital birth as they feel that they will be more comfortable with the emergency equipment close to hand, and may feel that they will receive more support in the first days immediately following the birth of their baby.

For similar reasons, other women opt for a Domino delivery. This includes a hospital birth with care provided by a familiar community midwife, but with a shorter stay in hospital.

Today more women are deciding on a home birth which is in my opinion the ideal environment, as the birth of your baby will occur as a normal part of family life and in an environment where ultimately you have the power to decide whom you want to attend the birth of your baby.

In all cases, you must decide on the right environment for you and discuss all the options with your partner and family to ensure their support before you make a decision.

At this point you may also like to consider whom you would like to support you during childbirth, and to witness the birth of your baby. This may not necessarily be the father of your baby, but could be your lover, friend, member of your family or another woman who has had an experience of childbirth.

You may also wish to have support from your aromatherapist. If you are planning a hospital birth it may be a good idea to obtain written permission from your consultant obstetrician to prevent any misunderstandings that could prevent your aromatherapist from attending you when you are admitted into your maternity unit.

YOUR FIRST ANTENATAL VISIT

Your first antenatal visit will take place shortly after your pregnancy is confirmed. This visit will give you a chance to meet some of the people who will be involved in your care during your pregnancy, such as your midwife, general practitioner or the staff involved in the running of the antenatal clinic at your local maternity hospital. This first visit will also give you an opportunity to discuss further your preferences for the type of care you would like during your pregnancy, and the environment in which you would prefer to give birth to your baby.

The type of physical examination you can expect will be very similar to that for preconceptual care. All the information concerning yourself and your partner is taken in complete confidence and recorded in your case notes. These case notes may be given to you for safe-keeping and, although they are the property of your local Health Authority, they are your responsibility until the birth of your baby and should be carried with you, especially if you are travelling away from home. This is because your case notes will document your progress throughout your pregnancy and will contain vital information should you require urgent treatment at another hospital.

It is of course up to you to decide who should be allowed to read your case notes, such as your family and friends, and they will be appreciated by your aromatherapist to share in your progress through your pregnancy.

SUBSEQUENT VISITS

At every antenatal visit you will be assessed physically by blood pressure estimation, urine tests and, in some centres, by measuring your weight gain throughout your pregnancy.

You will have your belly examined at each visit to assess the amount of liquor (fluid surrounding your baby), the growth of your baby, the position and heart beat and, in late pregnancy, whether the head has engaged (entered your pelvis) in preparation for birth.

In the first 28 weeks of your pregnancy you will be asked to attend monthly antenatal examinations. The frequency will then increase to fortnightly, and finally to weekly from week 36 until the birth.

At each visit you will be given time to discuss any problems or anxieties you may be experiencing, but by this point many women are overawed and leave without asking what they intended. Therefore it is always a good idea to jot down your questions on a piece of paper ready to ask at the end of your session before leaving the clinic.

6

SOME COMMON
DISCOMFORTS

This chapter describes some of the common discomforts that may affect you during the course of your pregnancy, and describes how aromatherapy can help relieve these conditions and promote natural healing.

On reading this chapter, your first impression may be that pregnancy is an unpleasant process and ill health increases with every passing week. This is not the case. Most women discover that pregnancy is in fact an incredibly enjoyable experience, making them both look and feel wonderful – a reflection of inner health.

Your own inner health is extremely important, for not only does it enhance your own feelings of well-being, but it will, to almost the same extent, have the same effects on the health and development of your baby.

Aromatherapy can be used in a variety of ways to induce relaxation, reduce tension and so much more to ensure that both you and your baby maintain this optimum inner health physically, mentally and spiritually.

Occasionally though, during pregnancy, even the healthiest woman may experience some common discomforts or ailments that, although considered minor in obstetric terms, are uncomfortable and will certainly affect your health and vitality. In fact if you are feeling generally unwell, pregnancy can become something that is endured rather than enjoyed, the approaching labour viewed with increasing apprehension, even dread, and the recovery following childbirth slow. But it also follows that if you are feeling healthy and full of energy, pregnancy becomes exciting, childbirth a challenge, and recovery rapid.

In the first few weeks of your pregnancy most of the discomforts that you may experience – fatigue, sickness and nausea – are caused on the whole by natural hormone changes. Aromatherapy will help you comfortably through these testing weeks until a natural hormone balance has been established, when these conditions usually resolve.

However, as your pregnancy advances, rising hormone levels that allow the relaxation and stretching of muscles and ligaments, together with pressure from the bulk and size of your rapidly developing baby, and changes in the shape of your body all have an effect, causing problems such as backache, constipation and circulatory disorders.

It is during this time that aromatherapy becomes invaluable. Used in a variety of ways in bath oils, compresses, massage and inhalations, essential oils provide fast and effective treatments in their own right, or they can be used to supplement most other therapies whether complementary or orthodox.

With the advance of modern medicine many have forgotten that pregnancy is a completely natural process and that medical intervention is not always necessary unless, of course, major problems develop. When used wisely, essential oils are completely safe and carry no danger of harming you or your baby – unlike some chemical treatments, whose harmful effects have sadly been clearly demonstrated in the past.

Do remember that if any of these common discomforts persist or become severe, or you experience a rise in body temperature, or if you suspect a change in your health generally, you must immediately seek further advice from those providing your professional care.

BACKACHE

You may experience some low back pain as your pregnancy advances. The reason for this is that, in order to compensate for your increasing weight and altered centre of gravity, you may develop an exaggerated curve in your back. The relaxation of muscles and ligaments within your pelvis in preparation for labour and birth may also contribute to this.

By regularly practising antenatal exercises you can help relieve some of the strain on overworked muscles. Try to rest for at least 15–20 minutes twice each day. Lying flat on your back on the floor, bend your knees up towards your chest, and resting your feet on a chair rotate your knees outwards. Next place a small rolled up towel, or a book, under your head, well away from your neck and shoulders, rest your arms by your sides, and relax (Figure 1). This position will help flatten out any exaggerated curves, as well as giving a good stretch along the whole length of your back.

Regular exercise in water will also help relieve the discomfort of back pain. Water not only gives support, but also helps tone and strengthen those back muscles affected by postural or hormonal changes. Try swimming or perhaps join an aquanatal group. These classes are available at most sports centres and consist of antenatal type exercises in water, and are particularly beneficial if you find 'land-based' exercise difficult. You may also find that postnatal exercise sessions in water will help your recovery following childbirth, and many centres offer 'duckling' classes for your baby to enjoy later.

I have found that most types of backache that develop in late pregnancy respond very quickly to massage with essential oils. Rosemary is particularly effective. This comforting essential oil has gentle warming properties that will increase your circulation and release tense or strained muscles. You can use Rosemary to help relieve any back pain you experience; apply as part of your self massage routine, or ask your partner to do this for you.

Rub the essential oil mixture over your lower back

using the flat of your hands. When your skin is well oiled, concentrate firmer pressure with the pads of your fingers or thumbs using deeper circular strokes. Massage until your muscles become warm and relaxed. Then to relax the muscles generally finish off with smooth lighter strokes with the flat of your hands, working over the whole area you have just treated (Figure 2).

If you feel that the pain is severe, rest and apply Rosemary in a warm compress. Place the compress over the area where you feel that the pain is centred, and cover the compress with a waterproof material to help retain the heat. Replace the compress as soon as it cools to body temperature.

This type of deep massage and Rosemary oil must not be

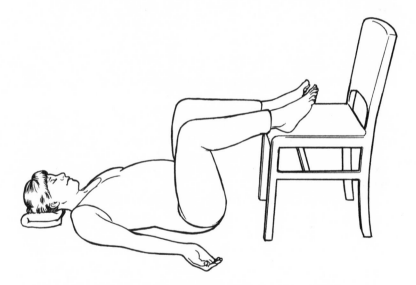

Fig. 1. Relaxation Exercise for Your Back

Lying flat on your back on the floor, bend your knees up towards your chest, rest your feet on a chair, and rotate your knees outwards. Place a small rolled-up towel, or a book, under your head, well away from your neck and shoulders. Rest your arms by your sides, palms uppermost. Relax.

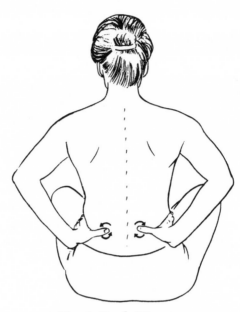

Fig. 2. Back Massage

Rub the essential oil mixture over your lower back using the flat of your hands. When your skin is well oiled concentrate firmer pressure with the pads of your fingers or thumbs, using deeper circular strokes.

used in early pregnancy, but can be safely used in the later weeks (from approximately 37 weeks onwards) when back pain is more likely to develop.

Occasionally some women find the heat generated by Rosemary oil rather uncomfortable. This is particularly common in the final weeks of pregnancy or during childbirth when you may already be feeling a little hot and bothered. In this case try Chamomile. This essential oil, which is safe to use in early pregnancy, can be applied in the same way as Rosemary, as a gentle back massage or in a warm compress. This subtle essential oil will help calm and reduce muscle spasm, as well as soothing and relaxing tension within the deeper muscle layers.

If possible, do try to receive a regular massage from your aromatherapist. These sessions will enhance your own treatments, and professionals who regularly practise massage will have the experience and confidence to work much deeper into the affected muscles.

Back Massage – Hints for Partners

Some people can naturally give a good massage, instinctively knowing where the aches and pains are felt and how much pressure to apply to relieve them. For most of us, though, massage is something that must be learned and practised.

If you are helping your partner through pregnancy and childbirth, being able to perform a good massage is perhaps one of your most important practical roles. Massage is not only a good way of applying essential oils, but also a very special way of communicating your love and support.

Of course, there is nothing to stop you massaging any part of the body during pregnancy. However, I feel that it is important for you to be able to perform a back massage particularly well as the back is the area where pain is most commonly experienced, especially in childbirth, and the strokes you will use can be adapted for any other part of the body. Also, the positions your partner will adopt for you to give the back massage are invaluable resting positions during labour, when they can easily be adapted to more upright positions to cope with the discomfort of contractions.

Before you begin, make sure that your partner is comfortable. For most pregnant women lying flat is uncomfortable, if not impossible. Sit your partner astride a chair leaning forward on to a pillow (Figure 3). Alternatively, place a towel or blanket on the floor or bed and help your partner into a kneeling position sitting back on her heels, knees well apart, and then help her to lean slowly forward from the hips to rest on several pillows or cushions (Figure 4). It is a good idea to ensure extra support by tucking a pillow under

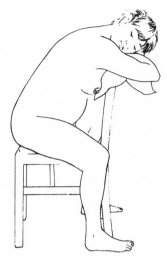

Fig. 3. Position for Back Massage (1)

Sit astride a chair, leaning forward on to a pillow.

her belly and another pillow over her heels and under her bottom to aid the circulation to her legs and prevent cramp developing. It is possible to massage the back with your partner lying on her side, but personally I find it difficult to apply an even pressure in this position.

Make sure you have everything to hand – massage oil and a blanket or towel. Remove any jewellery and wash your hands in warm water to ensure that they are not too cold. Pour a little massage oil into the palm of one hand, and then gently rub your hands together to warm and distribute the massage oil. This will ensure that your massage strokes will be smooth and even.

Place your hands flat on the lower back just below hip level. Then slowly slide your hands up the back on either side of the spine. Never massage over the bone as this can be painful. Move your hands up and across the shoulders, then down the whole length of the back. Continue this movement for several minutes until the back is well oiled and the muscles warmed. Now you can apply a firmer pressure

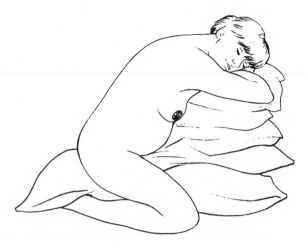

Fig. 4. Position for Back Massage (2)

Kneel on the floor, then slowly lean forward to rest on cushions or pillows. Gain extra support by tucking a pillow under your belly and another under your bottom to aid the circulation to your legs, thus preventing cramp.

to the areas that your partner finds painful. Use the heel of your hand or the pads of your fingers or thumbs. Concentrate on these areas using firm but gentle circular movements until you feel the muscles softening and relaxing.

Finish off your massage, using the same strokes you used at the beginning, to relax the back as a whole. Then cover the back with a blanket or towel to keep your partner warm, as oiled skin cools very quickly.

After giving your massage, allow your partner to rest for 5–10 minutes, or for as long as she is comfortable, before helping her to rise very slowly.

CIRCULATORY DISORDERS

As your pregnancy advances, the hormones that cause the relaxation of tissues associated with childbirth also cause a loss of tone in your blood vessels. This, together with the extra pressure of the weight of your growing baby, can cause extra strain on the arteries and veins of your lower belly causing circulatory disorders such as haemorrhoids, oedema (swelling), and varicose veins. Regular gentle exercise and resting with your legs raised, feet higher than hip level, will help stimulate your circulation, and by avoiding constipation you can prevent tissue damage on delicate blood vessels (see section on haemorrhoids p. 97).

Aromatherapy will provide valuable forms of therapy for both prevention and treatment of these conditions.

If you suffer from varicose veins, or have noticed them developing, you can treat them easily with essential oils. Cypress has the very special qualities of helping to heal and, at the same time, strengthen damaged tissue. Apply this essential oil diluted in carrier oil very gently over the areas affected by varicose veins taking care not to rub your skin as this friction can cause further damage. After applying a treatment, rest with your legs raised and allow the essential oil to be gradually absorbed.

There are many essential oils which, if applied frequently, will help tone and reduce the pressure within your circulatory system. Citrus oils, particularly Lemon, are especially effective in helping tone and stimulate sluggish circulation. For massage only a very low concentration is required as this essential oil has very powerful astringent qualities. Rosemary is another essential oil I occasionally recommend, but for use in late pregnancy only. Rosemary is valuable in helping stimulate the movement of fluids that accumulate within the tissues.

Try to give yourself a daily treatment with essential oils to relieve present problems, or if you feel that a build up of fluid is developing. Always make sure that you are comfortable before you begin your massage – in a position where you can easily reach your legs. Sitting on the floor is possibly the best.

If your feet are swollen, include them in your massage. Pour a little massage oil into the palm of one hand, and then gently rub your hands together to distribute the oil evenly. Apply a little massage oil to your feet, then begin by stroking from your toes up over your instep, then around your ankle. Then working on one leg at a time, apply a little more oil with smooth but firm strokes. With both hands circle your leg at the ankle and begin to pull up towards your knee using steady pressure, your thumbs sliding up the front bone, while your fingers apply a steady pressure behind your leg, massaging deep into the muscles.

Repeat this movement, massaging from ankle to knee several times to stimulate your circulation. Then, using each hand in turn, massage up your whole leg from ankle to knee, then from knee to groin. Always work with your circulation, massaging towards the heart.

Finish your massage by repeating the initial pulling strokes up your whole leg.

After your massage, rest with your legs raised up as high

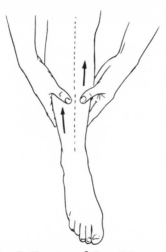

Fig. 5. Foot and Leg Massage

With both hands circle your leg at the ankle and begin to pull up towards your knee, using a steady pressure. Your thumbs slide up the bone at the front of your leg while your fingers apply steady pressure to the back of your leg, massaging deep into the muscles.

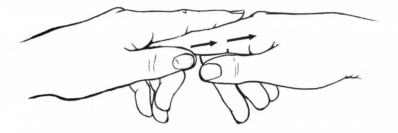

Fig. 6. Hand Massage

Rub oil into both hands. Using your forefinger and thumb grasp each finger in turn and massage using a 'stripping' action from the nail down towards the base of the finger.

as possible, either sitting or lying on the floor or in a chair with your feet resting on pillows or a low table. This position will support your aromatherapy treatments and help your circulation return to normal.

Remember never to massage directly over varicose veins, broken or infected skin. These areas must be treated separately.

Many women also suffer from swollen fingers and hands, especially during periods of hot weather. In this case use a little Lemon oil diluted in carrier oil for a quick hand massage.

Rub the oil into both hands. Then, using your forefinger and thumb, grasp each finger in turn and massage, using a 'stripping' action, down from your nail towards your finger base. Then briskly rub over your hand to your wrist, then from wrist towards your elbow. Repeat this massage again, working on each hand and forearm in turn.

Finish off by bending your arms at the elbows to raise your hands higher than shoulder level. Then alternately clench and open your hands in rapid succession several times. This action will help stimulate your circulation and drain the accumulated fluid.

At first you may not be aware of any visible difference following any of these treatments, but you may be assured that essential oils will continue to work long after your massage is complete.

CONSTIPATION

This uncomfortable condition can develop at any time, but is especially common in the last few weeks of pregnancy.

Unfortunately the same rising hormone levels that allow the relaxation of muscles and ligaments associated with pregnancy and childbirth also affect the muscular action of the large intestine. This causes a loss of tone and a sluggishness of movement along the digestive tract. Constipation can cause all kinds of aches and pains and a general lethargy that can be so acute that I have known some women so desperate to obtain relief that they have taken laxatives continuously throughout the entire course of their pregnancy! This is unfortunate because with slight adjustment to diet, exercise and regular treatments with essential oils, constipation can be prevented and the use of laxatives avoided – the long term use of which can cause lasting damage to the delicate tissues within the intestine.

If you have been prescribed iron supplements during your pregnancy, do make sure that these are absolutely necessary as they are often the cause of digestive upsets. I feel that today most women should be able to take an adequate diet, even when pregnant, and often these supplements are prescribed as a matter of course. If you believe that iron supplements are causing your problems, do discuss with your midwife whether these are really necessary. Often a change to a herbal preparation causes fewer problems.

Make sure that you eat plenty of foods that will add bulk and fibre to your diet – especially fresh fruit and vegetables – and drink large quantities of mineral or filtered water. Avoid eating too many dairy products and foods that are high in carbohydrates and sugar as these always make constipation much worse.

A regular massage with essential oils will help your digestion, and tone the muscles generally. Lavender has exceptionally energizing qualities and is effective in helping to increase the circulation and stimulate movement within your bowel. Use Lavender regularly, applying it as a back massage diluted 2 per cent in a carrier oil.

Position yourself comfortably, either sitting on a chair or on the floor, leaning forward slightly. Gently spread the oil over the whole area of your lower back, then concentrate your massage on areas that are particularly painful or tender to the touch. These symptoms indicate regions within your bowel that may be affected. Massage very gently using small circular strokes with the pads of your fingers or thumbs until you feel a reduction of tension or tenderness. Finish your massage with light strokes over the whole area using the flat of your hands.

A regular massage to the belly is also beneficial, increasing movement and flow along the bowel. Lying flat on the bed or floor, bend up your knees, keeping your feet flat on the floor. This position relaxes the muscles within the belly, making the massage more effective.

Apply the oil with gentle clockwise circular strokes over your whole belly. Then concentrate smaller deeper circular movements using your finger pads along the outer flank, remembering not to miss out the areas just above the hip bones on either side. Always work in a clockwise direction, and massage for just a few minutes only. Then finish off by using the same sweeping lighter clockwise strokes again over the whole belly. Finally, turn on to your side and rest for a few minutes before rising slowly.

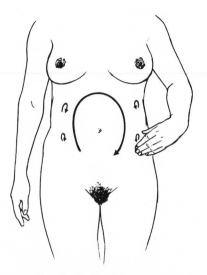

Fig. 7. Belly Massage

Apply the oil over the whole of your belly using gentle clock-wise circular strokes. Then concentrate smaller, firmer, circular movements using your finger pads along your outer flank.

Remember you must only perform this massage if you are happy doing so. Essential oils are very powerful. Go very gently, and if the massage becomes unduly painful stop, and seek further advice immediately.

INSOMNIA

During pregnancy sleep is often disturbed by the baby's movements, by having to get up frequently to pass urine, and through difficulty in finding a comfortable position.

I am always very aware of how most women become more anxious as their pregnancy advances. At this time, thoughts are dominated by their coming responsibilities as a parent, the hopes and fears for their baby and, of course, the approaching labour and birth. This is normal, although I firmly believe that it is vitally important for you to express these anxieties openly. Discuss them with your partner as well as those providing professional care. Surround yourself with individuals who are prepared to give you positive support. Listen to stories of good birth experiences – and ignore old wives tales.

I have found that it is during this time that aromatherapy comes into its own, boosting confidence, reassuring and comforting, and, most of all, increasing your ability to trust your body to follow what is after all a completely natural process.

Vaporize essential oils liberally around your home to promote a relaxing atmosphere. Before your bedtime relax in a warm aromatic bath, adding a few drops of your favourite essential oils. You may find the combination of Lavender and Chamomile especially good for easing away tensions, or perhaps the darker, earthier aromas of Sandalwood and Patchouli to boost confidence, or the more luxurious fragrances of Rose and Jasmine to celebrate your subtle feminine power. Most women discover that the experience of pregnancy and childbirth gives them a wonderful sense of achievement and feel much more confident in their own abilities and inner strength.

Sprinkle essential oils on to your bedding or nightclothes so that you can benefit from the healing vapours throughout the night. A regular massage with essential oils will reduce tension and induce relaxation – try giving yourself a daily massage or ask your partner to do this for you.

During your pregnancy your partner may also be experiencing similar conflicting emotions and a feeling of helplessness – particularly as men are at a biological disadvantage, not having the shared experience of being a woman. Most men find it difficult to truly appreciate the natural but dramatic physical and emotional changes taking place within you. Offer your partner the opportunity to give you practical support and also to share in your newfound knowledge of essential oils by giving him an aromatic massage so that he may also benefit from the healing powers of aromatherapy.

NAUSEA AND INDIGESTION

During pregnancy most women are affected by nausea, particularly in the first few weeks. This nausea and sometimes vomiting usually occurs in the morning, but can develop at any time during the day.

For many women the impact of the news of their pregnancy may cause a range of emotions from delight to intense apprehension. This is normal. But with this mixture of emotions and the imbalance of hormones that occurs in early pregnancy it is hardly surprising that you experience some kind of physical reaction. This I believe is nature's way of slowing you down during this period of rapid development.

Long ago our senses protected us from harm, and we depended on our natural instincts to survive. However, as we live our busy modern lives, these basic instincts are often neglected or most commonly ignored. During your pregnancy you should attempt to become more in tune with your body and aware of these protective mechanisms. This is vital for your own health and also that of your baby.

I am often approached by women who become very distressed during pregnancy, complaining of undue fatigue and nausea, or the sudden dislike of certain foods or odours. My usual advice is always to go with what your body is telling you.

If you are tired, try to sleep; if suffering from aches and pains, rest and your body will soon recover. Be sensible and avoid foods and odours that you find unpleasant. As these are most commonly alcohol, coffee, tea and tobacco, nature is certainly trying to protect you from these potentially harmful substances.

One great advantage of using aromatherapy during your

pregnancy is that essential oils will not interfere with your natural instincts, but can in fact enhance your awareness of them. I am certain that if you follow these natural instincts coming from within yourself, you and your baby will pass more comfortably and safely through pregnancy and childbirth.

Although most essential oils should be avoided during early pregnancy, Lavender if used with caution is perfectly safe and will help settle your stomach, and calm those feelings of panic and anxiety. Sprinkle a few drops on your bedding or nightclothes, or evaporate a little essential oil in your bedroom. Add a little Lavender oil to your bath each morning to feel refreshed and more able to face the day. I also advise some women to carry a little oil in a bottle or soaked into a cotton wool pad so that they can inhale the reassuring vapours if faced with any 'emergencies' during the day.

Nausea and indigestion may also develop in the later weeks of your pregnancy – often as the result of pressure on the stomach from the uterus which rises higher up your belly as your baby develops, and a relaxation of muscles that hold your stomach tightly closed between meals. Adapting your diet to exclude rich foods, tea and coffee may help reduce the feeling of nausea; while taking herb teas, such as Chamomile or Fennel, will help your digestion.

Although it must not be used in early pregnancy, Peppermint oil is very effective in helping relieve the nausea and indigestion of late pregnancy.

If indigestion develops, apply Peppermint as a massage. Rub it in lightly over your upper belly, or between your shoulder blades. If you feel that the indigestion is becoming severe, rest and apply the essential oil in a cold compress, regularly replacing the compress as soon as it warms to body temperature. If nausea develops, rest and use Peppermint in a cold compress over your forehead, or apply a little of the neat oil to your temples to calm your whole body. Many women also find these treatments useful in helping relieve the nausea that occasionally develops with the onset of labour, or during the later stages of childbirth. Lavender is reassuring and calming, while Peppermint helps clear the head and focus the mind. These essential oils do not, I feel, work well together but can be selected and applied according to your needs at that particular time.

CRAMP

This condition is common in late pregnancy and usually affects the muscles of the buttocks, thighs or lower leg. This is because these groups of muscles must work much harder during the later weeks of pregnancy to help support the extra load, especially the increasing weight of the uterus, and they can easily become over-tired. This fatigue may cause prolonged muscle spasm, which produces severe pain, usually at the end of the day or at night.

You may also suffer cramp during labour, especially if you stay in any position that will impede your circulation for too long – particularly positions such as kneeling or squatting.

Muscle cramp can also develop during your recovery following the birth of your baby. Most commonly this affects the muscles of the neck and shoulders, and is usually the result of muscle tension which may develop as you begin to establish breast-feeding your baby.

If you begin to suffer cramp during your pregnancy you will find that over-tired muscles respond well to the regular practice of simple yoga-type stretching exercises such as those taught in most antenatal classes.

Massage, especially with essential oils, will help to reduce muscle tension and increase circulation to tired muscles, as will slightly adjusting your diet to include more foods that are rich in salts and calcium, such as whole grains and green leafy vegetables, especially in periods of hot weather when cramp may become more of a problem.

During labour, try to stand occasionally, then stretch

and massage your legs. A brisk aromatic massage will help increase your circulation and prevent cramp developing.

Stand tall with one leg in front of the other, your hands flat against a wall at shoulder level. Ease your back leg further away from the wall and gently press your heel to the floor until you feel a stretch in your calf muscle. Hold this stretch for several seconds, then release. Now change legs. Repeat this stretch several times with each leg.

When you begin to breast feed it is important that you make sure that your back is well supported with cushions, and it may also help to have your baby raised slightly towards your breast by laying your baby on a pillow. This will help prevent unnecessary strain, and will help keep your neck and shoulder muscles relaxed.

In all cases you will find that regular massage with essential oils will do much to help reduce the likelihood of muscle cramp developing. All treatments are described in more detail in other sections of this book, the type of treatment being dependent on which muscle group is affected and at what stage of pregnancy and childbirth.

HEADACHES

During your pregnancy you may experience mild headaches. Headaches most commonly affect women during the early weeks of pregnancy when they are associated with early morning sickness, usually caused by hormonal changes, and are resolved once a natural hormonal balance is established. However, headaches may also develop in the later weeks of your pregnancy. These may be due to poor posture, fatigue or muscle tension particularly in the neck and shoulders.

In all these cases, headaches may be an important sign that you should pay special attention to your posture when standing or sitting, and that you must make more time to relax and rest as much as possible. Also, a slight adjustment to your diet may help reduce the chances of headaches developing or at least ease their severity. If you feel that you are susceptible to headaches, try excluding stimulants such as tea, coffee and, of course, alcohol and cigarettes. During their pregnancy many women also develop a heightened sensitivity to certain foods such as chocolate or dairy products. So if you do become affected by headaches, you may need to examine your diet for any substances that could be causing this type of allergic reaction.

Using aromatherapy will help you reduce the discomfort of headaches as well as help relieve the muscle tension that may be their cause.

As soon as you begin to experience a headache, try using a little Lavender oil, which if used with care is safe to use in early pregnancy. Apply one drop of neat Lavender oil to each temple using a cotton bud. Then, using your finger tips, gently massage the essential oil into your skin very slowly using small circular strokes.

Alternatively, use a little Lavender oil in a cold compress to your forehead. If you feel that your headache is the result of muscle tension, use Lavender diluted in a little carrier oil for a gentle massage to your neck and shoulders. You can do this yourself (see *self massage* p.70), or ask your partner to do this for you. Drink plenty of filtered or mineral water, and then, if it is possible, rest until you feel your headache improve.

If you are particularly troubled by headaches, or are at all concerned, do seek further advice immediately from your midwife.

7

MORE SERIOUS
PROBLEMS

Occasionally during pregnancy more serious problems may develop. But I believe that, as with any other disorder, if you maintain your everyday health during your pregnancy by eating a sensible diet and taking adequate amounts of rest and exercise, you will favourably influence the effects and ultimately the severity of these conditions.

Fortunately these serious problems respond extremely well to aromatherapy, if necessary combined with other prescribed treatments. Essential oils help reduce both the physical and emotional effects of illness, as well as boosting your body's own defences thus protecting you from further complications developing.

Before I go any further, however, it is important to stress that if you suspect a serious problem has developed, if you experience a rise in body temperature, or if you feel a change in your general health, you must seek further advice immediately. These conditions can rapidly affect your health and, in extreme cases, can impair the health and development of your baby.

If you have read the previous chapters you will be aware of how aromatherapy can help you maintain optimum health, as well as helping to relieve any minor disorders that may develop during your pregnancy. But it is in the event of more serious illness that you will really appreciate aromatherapy as a powerful treatment. Used in a variety of ways in baths, compresses, massage, local

washes and sitz-baths, essential oils will help promote healing and reduce discomfort, and will also supplement most
other prescribed treatments, complementary or orthodox,
by efficiently relieving the more serious effects of these
conditions and helping reduce the stress and anxiety that
usually accompany the development of physical illness.

It is now widely recognized that mental attitude will
influence a person's response to treatment – if you are
feeling depressed, tense or worried, recovery from illness
will take much longer. Using aromatherapy will help promote a positive mental attitude, which will keep you calm
and relaxed and allow your body to activate its natural
healing processes, thus ensuring a rapid improvement in
your condition and a speedy recovery.

One great advantage of using aromatherapy in your
treatment and recovery is its amazing versatility. You can
apply the essential oils in different ways that are appropriate
to each specific stage of your illness.

For instance, the onset of serious illness often causes a
rise in body temperature and a general malaise which
makes massage impossible; in this case apply essential oils
in compresses. Similarly, if you are confined to bed and
bathing is difficult, you can add essential oils to a local wash
instead. And do remember that if your condition makes it
impossible for you to use essential oils in any of the more
conventional methods you can always inhale the healing
vapours on blotting paper, or cotton wool, or even directly
from their bottles.

HIGH BLOOD PRESSURE

Throughout your pregnancy your blood pressure should
remain stable, although some women do develop high
blood pressure at this time. Research into this illness
continues as the cause is still not fully understood, but
if you do develop this condition, the best treatment you

can give yourself is rest and essential oils to keep you calm and relaxed.

Throughout your pregnancy it is important to be regularly examined by your midwife – not only to monitor your health and the development of your baby, but also to exclude the presence of high blood pressure. If detected and the condition is mild, you will be advised to relax at home, but in severe cases you may require hospital treatment for more observation of the effects of high blood pressure on you and your baby.

In both cases it is important that you improve your general health, and relax as much as possible. If your condition allows, give yourself a daily aromatherapy massage, or alternatively try regular visits to your aromatherapist, as a relaxing massage may help reduce your high blood pressure for several days. It is also important that you follow a sensible eating pattern.

Working as an independent midwife I have managed to achieve varying degrees of success by encouraging women affected by high blood pressure to follow a simple diet. This involves cutting out sugar, salt and stimulants such as tea, coffee, cigarettes and alcohol, reducing carbohydrates, and increasing the intake of potassium (found in foods such as bananas and tomatoes). This diet may not only help stabilize your blood pressure, but will certainly improve your general health and vitality.

Relax regularly in warm aromatic baths, and vaporize essential oils around your home to create a calming atmosphere. Lavender is particularly effective in times of stress and anxiety, or you can use other essential oils that you find restful. Favourites of mine include Chamomile, Frankincense and Neroli.

If you find that sleeping is difficult – a common condition in late pregnancy – sprinkle a few drops of essential oils on to your bedding or night clothes. The soothing effects will ensure a restful night.

You can also carry a few drops of essential oil in a bottle or soaked into a cotton wool pad so that you can regularly inhale the calming vapours. Many women find this method of using aromatherapy particularly useful when attending their maternity hospital for antenatal examinations which may be necessary should high blood pressure be diagnosed. Most women become quite anxious at this time, often fearing that the hospital visit will automatically result in admission to the antenatal ward for observation. This is not always the case, but with the stress and anxiety that a hospital visit may cause, the hustle and bustle of staff and visitors, as well as what is usually a long wait in the reception area, it is hardly surprising that your blood pressure may be raised by the time you are called to be examined.

If you do have to visit your local hospital antenatal clinic, find yourself a quiet place to rest and sit comfortably. Make sure that you have a few drops of essential oil handy to inhale regularly. Then, by the time of your consultation, your blood pressure will hopefully not be unduly affected.

It is interesting to wonder what the effects would be if essential oils were routinely vaporized in hospital waiting rooms, especially those of antenatal clinics. This simple procedure would not only make these institutions more pleasant places to visit and keep visitors relaxed, but aromatherapy might in fact reduce the number of patients admitted to the antenatal wards suffering from high blood pressure caused by the visit to the clinic itself rather than by pregnancy.

URINARY TRACT INFECTIONS

Urinary tract infections are uncomfortable and unpleasant. Common signs of infection are frequency in passing urine accompanied by pain just above the pubic bone or lower back.

During pregnancy you may become more susceptible to developing urinary tract infections for the hormones that influence the stretching of muscles and ligaments throughout pregnancy also cause a sagging of the vessels that convey urine to and from the bladder. This causes a pooling of fluid that can provide a breeding ground for bacteria. It is therefore important that you frequently flush your urinary system by drinking plenty of fluid, especially mineral or filtered water, and prevent bacteria from entering your system by regularly washing with unperfumed soaps.

The most common site of infection is the bladder, but in extreme cases infection can ascend as far as the kidneys. In this case your body will sense the development of a systemic infection and may begin premature labour, a mechanism designed to protect your vulnerable baby from the approaching bacteria. This can, however, be dangerous if your baby has not reached maturity. If you suspect a urinary tract infection has developed, it is therefore important that you seek further professional advice. Meanwhile you can immediately begin aromatherapy treatments. You can use a number of essential oils added to bidets, compresses, local washes or sitz-baths to help reduce discomfort, prevent a worsening of your condition, and encourage healing.

Bergamot is a light and refreshing essential oil which will help relieve the stinging and tenderness in the urinary opening. Sandalwood is particularly soothing if applied after passing urine when the discomfort can become more intense. You should add a few drops of the oil to boiled, cooled water and use as a local wash. Lavender is very effective in helping boost your body's defences, fight the infection and prevent the spread of bacteria within your urinary tract.

Drink plenty of fluid to flush your system, especially mineral or filtered water and fruit juice to dilute the concentrated urine. Fruit juice is often preferred when there is a loss of appetite as it will supply some of the natural sugars, minerals and vitamins so vital for your recovery.

You should rest as much as possible and, if the pain becomes acute, apply warm Chamomile compresses over the areas where pain is experienced. Chamomile will help reduce the discomfort of muscle spasm caused by irritation from the invading bacteria. Cover the compress with a waterproof material and replace as soon as it cools to body temperature.

If you are using antibiotics to treat your urinary tract infection you can still continue your aromatherapy treatments. But remember that as well as destroying harmful bacteria, antibiotics also reduce the natural organisms found within your body. These types of bacteria are part of your body's own defence system and help protect you from infection generally. Luckily these bacteria can easily be replaced by eating live yoghurt or by taking capsule supplements available at most health food shops.

VAGINAL INFECTIONS

During your pregnancy you may have an increased vaginal discharge. This is normal. But if you notice that this discharge changes in colour or odour, or if you experience itching of your vagina or vulva, an infection should be suspected. In this case aromatherapy treatments will immediately soothe the irritation, making you feel more able to cope with this uncomfortable condition, as well as helping to reduce the site of infection, prevent its spread, and encourage healing.

If you are receiving traditional treatments for your vaginal infection remember that you must apply essential oils before inserting the prescribed creams or vaginal pessaries. Essential oils are extremely efficient in helping treat vaginal infections and can be used singly or in combination, each essential oil having unique healing qualities. If you feel that the infection is acute, add a few drops to boiled then cooled water to use as a local wash, or simply add several drops to your bidet or sitz-bath and soak well.

Bergamot will help reduce inflammation and irritation within the infected areas, which for most women is the most distressing symptom of this infection. Using Ti-Tree will promote healing and help reduce the spread of infection. Both these essential oils work well when combined with Lavender. Lavender is always effective in combating infection and has all-round healing qualities that help reduce delicate tissue damage.

This condition responds well to treatment but, unfortunately, many women do suffer recurrent infections. You should take particular care to wash frequently using unperfumed soaps to reduce your chances of reinfection. A slight adjustment to your diet can also be effective, particularly avoiding tea, coffee and alcohol.

If you feel that you are particularly susceptible to vaginal infections, or are recovering from a previous infection, or if you are receiving antibiotic therapy, you must be extra vigilant.

8

CARRIER OILS

The carrier oils used to dilute essential oils prior to giving massage or applying topical treatments can be used to help prevent complications during childbirth.

Sometimes during pregnancy the baby will move into a breech (bottom first) position. Simple exercises and massage with carrier oils will help move the baby back into the normal head-first position. This will prevent the need for technically difficult procedures occasionally used to correct this malpresentation and reduce the chances of a potentially complicated labour and birth.

During the birth of your baby your perineum will stretch to a remarkable extent, but in spite of this elasticity it is frequently torn. Research has indicated that massaging your perineum with carrier oils will help prevent tearing or the need for episiotomy. (Episiotomy is a surgical incision used to enlarge the vaginal opening. A local anaesthetic solution is injected to numb the area, and then the cut, which extends from the vagina, usually diagonally, across through the perineum, is performed at the height of a contraction. This episiotomy is then sutured shortly after the birth under local anaesthetic.)

The carrier oil I usually recommend for both the following treatments is Sweet Almond oil, with a little added Wheatgerm oil for perineal massage if scar tissue is present.

The two following sections give full descriptions of how

carrier oils can be used for their own unique healing properties, as well as providing a base for essential oils.

BREECH POSITION

By the 36th week of your pregnancy, your baby should be lying in your uterus with their head down towards your pelvis in preparation for birth.

However, sometimes your baby will move, most commonly into a breech (bottom first) position. This may be due to a number of reasons such as the shape of your pelvis or uterus, or the growing site of the placenta. In these cases it is unwise to try and attempt to alter your baby's position.

Occasionally, though, your baby may move for no obvious reason. Mothers often associate this change with times of acute stress or anxiety. In these cases simple exercises and massage with carrier oils will help move your baby back into the normal head-first position, thus preventing the need for technically difficult procedures used occasionally by some obstetricians to attempt to correct this malpresentation, (known as external cephalic version which involves manually pushing the baby's head towards the feet until the head lies over the pelvis), and reducing the chances of a potentially complicated labour and childbirth.

Before you begin these exercises, do discuss them with your midwife to ensure that they are appropriate. Ask them to help you identify how your baby is lying, discovering the exact location of the head and spine. Also arrange to have an examination as soon as you suspect that your baby has moved, so that you can perform squatting exercises immediately in order to help your baby's head engage inside your pelvis.

Using the floor as a firm surface, adopt an all-fours position, and then slowly lower your chest to the floor (Figure 8). The object of this exercise is to position your hips on a level higher than your head.

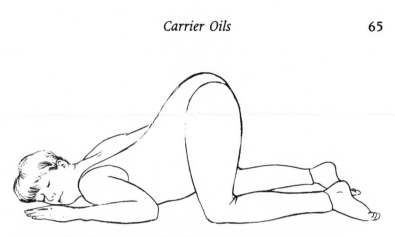

Fig. 8. Exercise for the Breech Position (1)

Adopt an all-fours position, then slowly lower your chest to the floor.

Alternatively, lie on your back with your hips raised high on pillows or cushions keeping your shoulders flat on the floor (Figure 9). When you are in position, use a little carrier oil to massage your belly over the area of your baby's back using a firm but gentle pressure. Try to stay in this position for 10–15 minutes at a time. You may need to perform this exercise several times each day, perhaps over

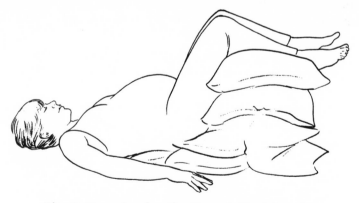

Fig. 9. Exercise for the Breech Position (2)

Lie on your back with your hips raised high on pillows or cushions. Keep your shoulders flat on the floor.

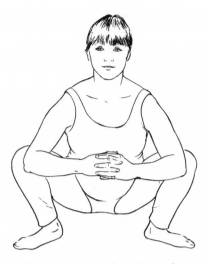

Fig. 10. Squatting Exercise

Keeping your back straight and your feet flat on the floor, slowly lower your bottom. Clasp your hands together and spread your knees apart with your elbows.

a period of many days before you feel your baby move. This is often described by mothers as a rapid movement or churning as the baby shifts position. If you believe that your baby has moved back into a head-first position, have this confirmed by your midwife. If you have been successful practise some squatting exercises.

Stand with your feet 2–3 feet apart, toes pointing forward. Keeping your back straight and feet flat, lower your bottom towards the floor, going down as low as possible. Then clasp your hands together and spread your knees apart with your elbows. If you find it difficult to keep your balance, hold on to a strong piece of furniture such as a door handle or radiator. Hold this position for a few minutes or for as long as you are comfortable. If you are suffering from varicose veins or haemorrhoids avoid very deep squatting exercises by supporting your bottom with books or a low stool.

When practised several times each day, this squatting

position will help to stretch your pelvic muscles and ligaments. This increases your pelvic opening, allowing your baby to move downward to help stabilize its position deep inside your pelvis.

PERINEAL MASSAGE

Your perineum will stretch to a remarkable extent during the birth of your baby, but in spite of this elasticity it is frequently torn. In extreme cases of either failure of your perineum to stretch or signs that a bad tear will develop, your midwife may need to perform an episiotomy. Research has shown that massaging your perineum daily for 5–10 minutes in the last 6 weeks of your pregnancy will help prevent tearing or the need for episiotomy.

Before you begin, make sure that your bladder is empty, wash your hands, then ensure that you are propped up comfortably. When first starting you might find that a warm bath will help stretch the tissues. Select a nut-based carrier oil such as Almond oil, adding a little Wheatgerm oil if you have any scar tissue from previous tears or episiotomy, as this oil will nourish damaged tissue and encourage elasticity.

Massage the carrier oil into your perineum and lower vaginal wall. Pay special attention to any scar tissue. Then place both your thumbs inside your vagina and press downwards towards your rectum. Maintaining a steady pressure move your thumbs along in a 'U' type of movement. Hold this stretch for 30–60 seconds, then release. Massage with more oil, stretch again to the maximum, hold, then release.

During your massage try to stretch your vaginal opening until you feel a burning or tingling inside your muscles. This sensation is similar to what you will experience when your baby's head begins to crown. At this point draw up your pelvic floor muscles, the muscles you would normally tighten when you try to stop urinating mid-stream, and feel how much more painful this sensation becomes.

It is by consciously relaxing your pelvic floor muscles during the moment of birth that you will also help prevent further tissue damage.

At first you may find it difficult to relax your pelvic floor muscles consciously, but the moment you experience this tingling or burning sensation during your perineal massage try to relax your muscles. Really concentrate and remember not to hold your breath, but continue breathing regular breaths in and out.

When you first begin practising perineal massage your tissues will feel tight, but with time and practice they will relax and stretch. Perineal massage should not be painful. If you do experience any problems do not hesitate to seek further advice.

9

LOOKING AFTER
YOURSELF

PAMPERING

Throughout your pregnancy you must take an active role in looking after yourself, developing a holistic approach to your health by continuously assessing your needs and those of your baby.

But pregnancy is also a time for pampering, and what better way than with aromatherapy? For, as you will discover, aromatherapy is not just a treatment for specific conditions – it is also a pleasurable experience. So enjoy yourself!

Why not liberally vaporize combinations of exotic essential oils around your home, or use a few drops for a warm aromatic bath. My own favourites include Lavender and Mandarin to start the day feeling fully awake and refreshed, Patchouli and Orange which to my mind possess the strength of the earth and the warmth of the sun, and Lemon and Frankincense to clear the mind and help focus the thoughts.

Having a regular massage with essential oils will help keep your skin soft, supple and looking radiant. Unfortunately I am not aware of any treatments that will prevent stretch marks, but Neroli will help nourish growing skin, and massage improves tone and elasticity.

Very often women complain that during pregnancy their hair becomes dry or dull. Condition your hair with essential oils. Use Rosemary to bring lustre to dark hair, or

Chamomile to lighten and add volume to fair hair. Add these essential oils to a final rinse after shampooing. You can also improve the condition of your hair by regularly giving your scalp a good brisk massage (see *Scalp Massage* p.79) and adding a little oil for extra shine.

By the end of your pregnancy you will probably have gained the equivalent of two bags of shopping in weight. This is quite a load to carry 24 hours a day! With so much going on in other parts of your body you may forget that pregnancy subjects your feet to all kinds of extra strain, and may assume that your feet can take care of themselves. In fact, caring for your feet during pregnancy as well as at other times can prevent many foot complaints developing in later life. Pamper your feet with aromatic foot baths. Fill a bowl with tepid water, then add a few drops of essential oils. Use Peppermint oil to cool and refresh the skin, or Cypress if your feet are particularly hot and perspiring, as pregnancy can increase the action of the sweat glands. Soak for 5–10 minutes. Gently pat your feet dry and then use a little essential oil for a special foot massage (see p.73). In order to experience the refreshing effects on your whole body, concentrate on areas that feel especially painful as these sites indicate poor circulation or tension.

SELF MASSAGE

Self massage is a really good way of getting to know your body and helping you become aware of the subtle as well as the dramatic changes that will occur during your pregnancy. For pregnancy is much more than just the development of your baby. Pregnancy is an event that will affect the whole of your body. But don't worry. These changes, caused by increasing hormone production, circulation and metabolism are completely natural, and are necessary in order to support your baby through the months of rapid growth, to prepare your body for labour and childbirth, and to help you cope with the demands of feeding and caring for your baby.

It is worth your while trying to become familiar with these changes for not only will this make you more aware of what to expect, but in many ways help you understand why you look and in part why you feel the way you do at each stage of your pregnancy.

Even as early as 3 weeks into your pregnancy you may begin to look and feel different. You may notice a tingling or a sensation of fullness in your breasts, or may be affected by nausea and vomiting, due to rising hormone levels. Perhaps you may also be aware of having to pass urine frequently due to pressure on your bladder from your growing uterus.

By 12 weeks you may be able to palpate your uterus just above your pubic bone. This is the time when you may become aware of some skin changes, such as darkening of your nipples, areola, and face, and a fine dark line may appear which extends from your pubic bone up to your umbilicus, again due to an increase in hormone production.

A few weeks later your breasts will become enlarged and begin to secrete colostrum which will continue throughout your pregnancy until you begin to breast feed and produce milk. This ensures that all milk ducts are potent, so that fluid can flow freely when you begin to feed your baby.

By 18 weeks you may experience your baby's first fluttering movements, and 4 weeks later be able to recognize limbs, hands and feet. At this time the heart beat can be heard clearly when an ear is placed to your belly over the area where your baby is settled.

Slowly your size and shape will begin to change as increasing hormone levels stimulate the growth of your uterus and breasts, and cause a relaxation of muscles and ligaments in preparation for labour and birth. Now you are breathing for two, and your lower ribs expand outwards so that you can take in slower deeper breaths. Even your own heart beats a little faster and becomes stronger as the muscles pump up to 40 per cent more blood around your body, to feed and nourish your baby.

These are only a few of the changes that will take place very gradually over several weeks and months. Giving yourself a regular massage will help you become familiar with and proud of your changing body, as well as help you monitor or detect any problem areas that may exist or develop, such as oedema, varicose veins or stretch marks, so that you can begin to use aromatherapy treatments immediately.

You can of course give yourself a quick massage at any time of the day – while at work, when travelling, or even in the waiting room of your antenatal clinic. But I believe that it is important that you occasionally give yourself time to get fully acquainted with your changing self, to rest, and to spend some time in special communication with your baby who will enjoy your massage as much as you will.

Prepare your massage oil before you start. Use a nut-based carrier oil that is easily absorbed by your skin. Add a little Wheatgerm oil if your skin is dull or dry, and a few drops of the essential oils of your choice. Perhaps Lavender for all-round therapeutic qualities, Mandarin to refresh and renew energy, Chamomile to soothe and induce relaxation, or Neroli to nourish growing skin.

Find yourself a warm peaceful room where you know you will not be disturbed. You can give your massage sitting on your bed, but usually the floor provides a firmer surface. Sit on a soft blanket or towel.

If possible, before you start your massage, undress and stand in front of a full-length mirror so that you can closely observe your body, and easily recognize changes in your body shape or posture. These changes can often be corrected by exercise or massage, or by paying more attention to the way you stand or sit. This way you can avoid unnecessary aches and pains by trying to carry the extra weight and bulk of your uterus in the centre of your body, described by some mothers as rather like trying to balance an egg (your uterus) in an egg cup (your pelvis).

Once you are comfortable, begin your massage. There is no particular order you should follow, but you will find it more relaxing if you develop a routine by working up from your feet to your head, so that your massage becomes instinctive, concentrating on the areas that feel tense or tired.

Feet and Legs

Sitting down, work on each foot in turn. Using both hands smooth a little massage oil over your whole foot. Then

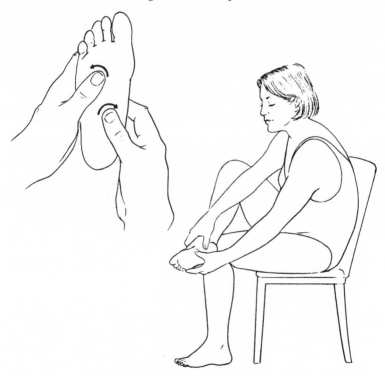

Fig. 11. Foot Massage

Concentrate on the sole of your foot, working over the entire area with small circular movements using your thumbs or finger pads.

concentrate on the sole of your foot, working over the entire area with small circular movements using your thumbs or finger pads. Then stroke, rotate and pull each toe in turn. Finish off by massaging over your whole foot again, then up and around your ankle. Stroke up your lower leg to your knee, then stroke up the upper leg, always massaging towards your heart.

Hips

Lying on your side, bend your knees towards your chest. Massage with firm but gentle strokes around your whole hip from the front bones of your pelvis, round your hip and over your buttocks. Then roll on to your other side and repeat.

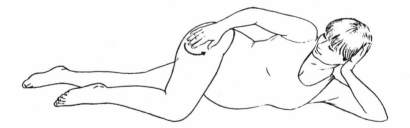

Fig. 12. Hip Massage

Lying on your side, bend your knees towards your chest. Massage around the whole hip with firm but gentle strokes.

Lower Back

Sitting down, apply a little massage oil to your lower back using the flat of your hands to warm the muscles. Now

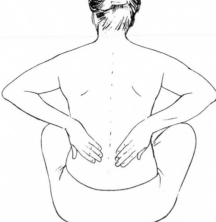

Fig. 13. Lower Back Massage

Apply a little massage oil to your lower back using the flat of your hands. Then concentrate a firmer pressure on the more painful areas using your thumb or finger pads to release tight muscles.

concentrate a firmer pressure on the more painful areas using your thumbs or finger pads to release tight muscles. Finish off by gently stroking the whole area to relax the muscles generally.

Chest

There is no massage that will prepare your breasts for feeding, but massaging your whole chest area will improve your circulation and the quality of your skin. Massage gently over your chest area working from your collar bone down and over your breasts, then out and down between your ribs.

Arms and Hands

Massage one hand then arm at a time. Gently stroke a little oil over your hand. Stretch, rotate, then pull each finger. Smooth over your hand then up your arm, over your elbow to your shoulder.

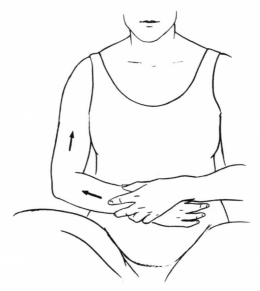

Fig. 14. Arm and Hand Massage

Massage one hand and arm at a time. Gently stroke a little oil over your hand. Stretch, rotate, then pull each finger. Smooth over your hand then up your arm, over your elbow to your shoulder.

Shoulders and Neck

You can massage these areas either sitting up or lying down, depending on how comfortable you feel in either position.

Using a little massage oil, begin to work on one side of your neck and shoulders at a time using the flat of the opposite hand. Press, then massage using light circular strokes over the whole area. Then using a firmer pressure,

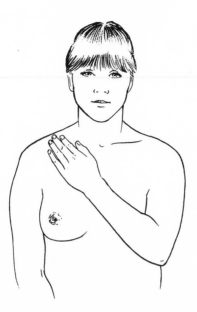

Fig. 15. Shoulder and Neck Massage

Using a little massage oil, work on one side of your neck and
shoulders at a time, using the flat of the opposite hand. Massage
using light circular strokes over the whole area, then, using a
firmer pressure, work on any tense or knotted muscles using
finger pads and thumb.

work on any tense or knotted muscles using finger pads
and thumb, gently pinching and kneading these muscles.
Finish off by using the same circular strokes you used at
the beginning, massaging the sides and back of your neck,
and as much of the upper back as you can reach comfortably
without straining.

Face

Using a small amount of massage oil, smooth across your
forehead with your fingertips. Always use both hands
together to keep your massage symmetrical. Work from

the inside out, starting at the hairline down towards the arch of your eyebrows. Then stroke down the sides of your face, up and over your cheek bones to your nose, down and around your mouth. Repeat this movement several times.

Now work on your jawline. Using both hands, hold your jaw at your chin, then move your hands apart, using pinching movements along the bone out towards your ears. Massage gently along the bone several times, until you feel the muscles soften and relax.

To finish, use the flat of your hands to stroke down the whole of your face in one continuous movement, beginning at your forehead, over your eyes, nose and mouth, along your jawbone down to the base of your neck. Repeat this stroke again. This helps 'connect' the different areas that you have been working on as well as relaxing the facial muscles as a whole.

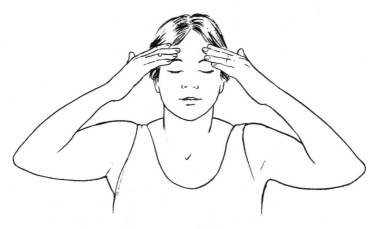

Fig. 16. Face Massage

Using a small amount of massage oil, smooth across your forehead with your finger tips. Use both hands together to keep your massage symmetrical. Work from the centre out, starting at the hairline and moving down towards the arch of your eyebrows. Then stroke down the sides of your face, up and over your cheek bones to your nose, down and around your mouth. Repeat several times.

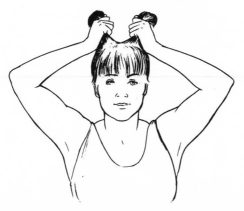

Fig. 17. Scalp Massage – pulling the hair

Taking a bunch of hair at a time, gently rotate and pull, working over the entire area of the scalp.

Scalp

Using both hands, spread out your fingers over your head and, with your finger pads, begin to move your scalp. Concentrate on areas of your scalp where the muscles feel tight and do not move freely. Then, using your finger pads again, rub the skin briskly. Now take a bunch of hair at a time and gently rotate and pull, working over the entire area of the scalp. Finish by stroking over your scalp using first your finger pads, then the flat of alternate hands, your strokes becoming lighter and lighter, gently relaxing all the connecting muscles and tissues.

Belly

Try lying flat on your back, but if this is difficult bend up your knees, keeping your feet flat on the floor. Using a little oil, massage your whole belly very gently with circular clockwise strokes.

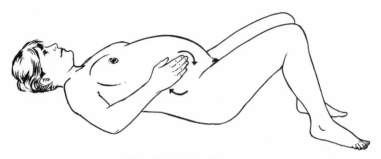

Fig. 18. Belly Massage

Lie on your back – if necessary bend your knees, but keep your feet flat on the floor. Using a little oil, massage your whole belly very gently with circular clockwise strokes.

After giving yourself a full body massage you should be completely relaxed. Cover yourself with a soft blanket or towel and make yourself comfortable lying on your side. Then rest.

Often during massage baby likes to join in, pushing out limbs for you to massage. This forms a good basis for baby massage after birth. Most mothers report that their babies become much calmer, perhaps lulled to sleep by the rhythmic massage strokes and the relaxing effects of massage with essential oils experienced by their mothers.

10

THE BIRTH

Childbirth is a very demanding process. Good preparation is the key to helping to cope as well as possible, and to take an active role in giving birth to your baby.

It is important that during your pregnancy you try to understand the processes involved in childbirth by joining an antenatal class or birth group so that you are aware of what to expect at each stage of labour and birth. Following an exercise programme such as antenatal exercises, swimming and walking will increase your stamina and strengthen the muscles involved during the birth process.

If you are planning to give birth to your baby in hospital try to become familiar with your maternity unit, and if possible try to meet the midwives who work in that department. This meeting will provide a good opportunity to involve the staff in your progress during your pregnancy, to discuss with them any aromatherapy treatments you propose to use, as well as any apprehensions you may be experiencing.

Fears and anxieties concerning labour and childbirth are normal. But if you are worried or lacking in confidence in yourself or your supporters, you may soon begin to feel isolated, or feel that your care is being in some way dictated to you and that you are beginning to lose control over events. This is not only very distressing in itself but will also make it very difficult for you to cope with the emotional as well as the very physical demands of childbirth, and can in fact affect your progress through each stage. Open discussion will help calm these emotions, promote a positive and optimistic attitude as well as greater confidence in those providing your professional care.

When labour begins, many women fear that the intense pressure of the contractions will in some way distress their baby. Certainly if you are receiving chemical treatments such as those needed to induce labour or to relieve discomfort, you and your baby must be monitored closely to make sure that all is well. But I believe that most babies in fact enjoy the process of birth, as the increasing strength and frequency of contractions prepares them for independence by stimulating muscles and circulation as well as providing the opportunity to stretch more freely as they move down the birth canal.

It is important that you continue to use aromatherapy to help support you and your baby both physically and emotionally, for essential oils will help relieve discomfort as well as promote relaxation. Remember that if you remain calm and relaxed so too will your baby to almost the same extent.

Make sure that your birth partner is familiar with how to use each essential oil that you intend to use during the birth as they will be responsible for preparing and applying each treatment as you require it, for it will be very difficult for you to apply your own. You can also ask your midwife to help if you experience difficulties. As labour begins, you will become totally committed to the birth of your baby, perhaps oblivious of your surroundings, even your supporters, allowing you the freedom to follow your own natural instincts and your body's natural processes.

THE ROLE OF YOUR BIRTH PARTNER

Supporting a woman through childbirth is an incredibly rewarding experience, but an extremely demanding role which unfortunately many birth partners approach knowing very little about what is expected of them.

Your birth partner may not necessarily be the father of your baby, but someone who you feel will be the best person to support you during this important time, preferably someone who will be available to give you support during your pregnancy and become involved in the development of your baby.

During your pregnancy you must encourage your birth partner to become familiar with the events of pregnancy and the processes of childbirth in preparation for their important role of supporting you during the birth itself.

Most antenatal programmes run couples' evenings when birth partners are invited. Ask your partner to attend with you if they are unable to join at any other time. These sessions focus on the various ways that a baby may be born, the role of the birth partner, and what will be expected of them during your labour and the birth of your baby. Your birth partner will also have an opportunity to talk to other individuals who have been asked to give similar support, and share their hopes and concerns if they wish.

If possible, it is also a good idea for your birth partner to attend your antenatal clinic with you occasionally, especially if you are planning a hospital birth. These visits will help them become familiar with the hospital and staff.

Most maternity units also offer tours of the maternity department and the areas where labour and birth will take place. This visit will not only help reduce the fear of the unknown, but will give the opportunity for your birth partner to become familiar with the route to your hospital and parking facilities if they are going to be responsible for transporting you to hospital when labour begins. As you prepare for childbirth you must decide through discussion with your birth partner how they are going to participate.

Unfortunately this shared experience can lead to natural feelings of helplessness, especially if your partner is likely to become distressed at the sight of you in pain. Beware of making any 'pacts' with your birth partner.

I have heard of women anxious to avoid artificial methods of pain relief, make their birth partner promise to prevent them from succumbing when contractions become painful. The best plan you can make is to take each stage at a time and avoid putting your birth partner in this difficult situation. Remember that decisions concerning your care during childbirth are ultimately yours, and only you know how you really feel at each stage of your labour.

As the time for the birth of your baby draws nearer make sure that your birth partner is freely available to attend you at any time, can be easily contacted and is familiar with your maternity hospital phone numbers in case they should have to telephone on your behalf once labour begins.

If you are planning for a water birth, make sure that your birth partner is capable of constructing, filling and emptying the pool. It will also be their responsibility to ensure that the correct water temperature is maintained when you use the pool for labour and giving birth to your baby.

If you are intending to use aromatherapy treatments during childbirth, your birth partner must know which essential oils you propose to use and how to prepare and apply them. It is also a good idea for them to practise massage techniques with you well beforehand (see *back massage* pp. 38 ff.) as well as becoming familiar with the position you would prefer to use to help you cope with contractions, and the positions you would like to adopt to give birth to your baby.

If necessary you may like to visit your aromatherapist with your birth partner should you feel that you need further advice concerning the use of essential oils and massage techniques for childbirth. Your birth partner may also benefit from aromatherapy treatments if they are feeling particularly stressed by natural fears and anxieties – you must remember that most birth partners feel under a great deal of pressure to live up to your expectations.

Do discuss all your apprehensions openly and honestly. Give your permission beforehand so that your birth partner is free to leave the birth place at any time either for fresh air or food, or if they feel that they cannot be present for the actual birth of your baby.

If you are planning a home birth you are totally in

control and can decide who you wish to have with you during childbirth. But birth partners are always welcome in maternity units for your midwife cannot always be in constant attendance, particularly in the early stages of labour.

You will find that your birth partner will have a reassuring and calming presence, particularly in the case of a hospital birth when, unfortunately, they may be the only familiar face whispering words of encouragement, offering cool drinks of water, trying to make you as comfortable as possible with aromatic massage, while still respecting your space as you use all your energy to cope with stronger contractions. Your birth partner, acting as a buffer between you and your surrounding environment, will help maintain a calm and peaceful atmosphere by reducing unnecessary intrusions.

The mother and her birth partner have a very special relationship which develops through the shared experience of childbirth, an experience I have been privileged to share on many occasions working as a midwife, aromatherapist and friend.

WHAT TO TAKE INTO HOSPITAL

If you are planning a home birth you will hopefully have everything to hand as long as you have carefully prepared your equipment beforehand.

If you have decided to give birth in hospital you must be well organized to take everything that you will need with you, to prepare and use your aromatherapy treatments, and to make you as comfortable as possible. I suggest that you pack the items you may need for labour and childbirth in a separate bag.

- a large comfortable nightshirt/shirt/pyjama jacket
- a pair of warm socks
- a bean bag or large pillow if these are not supplied by your hospital

- mineral water (the bottle can be used later to prepare aromatic local washes)
- carrier oil
- essential oils and an essential oil burner or aromatherapy fan
- a saucer or shallow dish for mixing massage preparations
- flannels and small towels to make compresses
- waterproof material to cover compresses
- food for your birth partner.

Your midwife will tell you what you will need for yourself and your baby after the birth.

INDUCTION OF LABOUR

When planning for the birth of your baby you must remember that the birth date calculated from the first day of your last menstrual period is approximate and the actual birthdate can vary by days or even weeks.

Occasionally when it does not begin spontaneously, labour may be induced by procedures that include the use of synthetic hormones, usually administered in the form of vaginal pessaries or intravenous infusions, and by artificially rupturing the membranes which surround your baby.

Some women attempt to induce labour by taking hot spicy foods, by taking laxatives such as castor oil (50 per cent castor oil/50 per cent orange juice in a tumbler size glass), and by sexual intercourse. But if you are considering trying these methods, do discuss them with your midwife first to make sure that they are appropriate. These methods are often successful but I do not suggest that you try all three at the same time!

One equally successful but more gentle method that I occasionally recommend to induce labour, is with essential oils. Use Clary Sage for a belly massage twice each day. Massage firmly but gently with circular clockwise strokes for 5–10 minutes. Then add a few drops of Clary Sage to a warm bath each evening to ensure a good night's sleep which will leave you feeling much more refreshed and able to cope when labour does eventually start.

LABOUR

If you have been fortunate enough to remain fit and well during your pregnancy you may have had no more than a passing interest in aromatherapy. But I am certain that you will appreciate the value of aromatherapy during your labour and the birth of your baby as essential oils help relieve most of the physical discomforts and emotional anxieties that you may experience.

It is always very exciting when labour first begins, realizing that your pregnancy is almost at an end and that at last you will soon be welcoming your baby into your world. But do try to remain calm and relaxed. One good way is by vaporizing a little of your favourite essential oils to help you focus your thoughts and energies while you make those final preparations.

When your contractions become stronger, concentrate on your natural instincts for comfort, conserve your energy, and rest as much as possible. At this point you will find a warm aromatic bath very soothing.

As labour advances, lying flat is very uncomfortable for most women. Try either sitting astride a chair leaning forward on to a pillow or, alternatively, a kneeling position with your knees relaxed apart, leaning forward from your hips to rest on pillows or a bean bag if you have one. For extra support tuck a pillow under your belly with another pillow under your bottom to aid the circulation to your legs. I have found that for most women, these provide valuable resting positions and you will find it very easy to move into more upright positions to help you breathe through stronger contractions.

While resting, use essential oils for a gentle massage over your shoulders, back, hips and legs, concentrating a firmer pressure on particularly painful areas.

For more intensive treatment, use essential oils in a warm compress. Most women find this comforting especially if they are experiencing discomfort in the lower back. Cover the compress with a waterproof material to help retain the heat, and replace it as soon as it cools to body temperature.

Occasionally stand and stretch out your legs to prevent cramp developing. If necessary stimulate your circulation by using a little essential oil for a brisk massage, working up your legs and always massaging towards your heart, to help your circulation quickly return to normal.

If you have used aromatherapy throughout your pregnancy, you will by now have your own favourites to suit each mood.

During childbirth you may find that, like most women, you experience several changes in mood from elation to despair, laughter to tears. This is normal. One of the great advantages of using aromatherapy to support you during labour is that you can select the essential oil to complement your emotions: Lavender to induce relaxation, Chamomile to release inner tensions, Bergamot or Mandarin to renew energy, Rose or Jasmine to reassure and boost confidence.

Occasionally I use Clary Sage during labour. This essential oil has a very special action of toning the muscles of the uterus and is particularly effective if your contractions are weak or irregular and progress towards the birth of your baby is slow. If this is the case, find a comfortable position either sitting upright on a chair, or on the bed well supported by pillows. Apply a little Clary Sage to your belly between contractions using circular clockwise strokes, applying a firm but gentle pressure using the flat of the hands. Concentrate on relaxing the muscles of your lower belly allowing your baby to move downward to press firmly on the neck of your uterus. This pressure will help your uterus open and, in turn, stimulate further contractions.

Continue this massage for 10–15 minutes or until regular contractions are established.

Clary Sage should only be used after discussion with your midwife to make sure that it is appropriate and that your slow progress is not due to any cause other than ineffective uterine action.

EPIDURAL ANAESTHETIC

If you decide to have an epidural anaesthetic during labour (a form of pain relief using a local anaesthetic solution injected into your back using a fine cannula) you can still continue aromatherapy.

Although you will be surrounded by the drips and monitors needed whenever this type of medication is given, you can still receive massage of your hands, face and feet. This gentle massage with essential oils is both comforting and healing and will help relieve tension and lessen the feeling of isolation that many women experience who are confined to bed, as this form of pain relief demands.

WATER BIRTH

If you are intending to give birth to your baby in water, remember to remove all traces of essential oils before you enter the water of the birthing pool. This can be done quickly and easily using a mild soap and water solution.

CHARGING THE ATMOSPHERE

If massage is inappropriate, as in the cases of preparation for birth by Caesarean section or water birth, or if you wish to enhance your environment generally, vaporize a few drops of essential oils to quickly charge the atmosphere.

Evaporate essential oils in essential oil burners or vaporizers; but do check that these are allowed if you are planning to use them in your maternity unit, as most hospitals have strict rules regarding the lighting of candles or powering of electrical equipment. If it is not possible for you to use these appliances, essential oils can be rapidly vaporized by adding several drops to a bowl of hot water, the surface of a warm radiator or the bulb of a bedside lamp before switching on.

IMMEDIATELY FOLLOWING THE BIRTH

During the first moments following the birth of your baby you will probably experience a surge of energy and emotion, no matter how fatigued or even totally exhausted you have felt moments before the birth.

The events immediately following the birth are very intimate. This is a time during which you can get to know your baby, and your baby slowly begins to adjust to the new environment and becomes familiar with your smell, the shape of your face and to recognize the sound of your voice.

During this time you and your baby will feel extremely sensitive. It is therefore important that noise is kept to a minimum and that the lighting in the birth room is dimmed and your baby is kept warm and comfortable against your bare skin. Even if the birth has been difficult or complicated by forceps or Caesarean section, this atmosphere can easily be created quite quickly after the birth.

Initially most mothers spend time just looking at and holding their baby. When your baby shows signs that they are ready and you are comfortable you can begin to breast feed.

It is good to begin to breast feed as soon as possible after the birth as the instinctive sucking reflex is likely to be strong – although you may find that your baby just needs to rest at first and will lie peacefully in your arms, especially if you have experienced a long labour, or your baby a difficult birth. Then you will both need rest, and your baby will need gentle body contact for reassurance.

Later, after feeding, you will be able to wash and dress your baby. Your midwife or birth partner can help you do this or, if facilities allow, you may like to have a bath with your baby, soaking in comfortable warm water; or you may wish to give your baby a soothing massage using a plain carrier oil. As it is not really necessary to bath your baby immediately, you may prefer to wait for the vernix (the white greasy substance on your baby's skin) to be absorbed which will help protect the skin and keep it soft and supple.

While you leave your baby to sleep you can take time to wash and change and apply any aromatherapy treatments that you feel are necessary.

The period of bonding with your baby may vary and can last minutes or several hours but, above all, it should be an experience that is gentle and caring while you, your partner, and your baby spend some time together undisturbed.

11

RECOVERY

The first few days, weeks and months following the birth of your baby should be a time when you slowly develop your confidence and independence, during which a strong bond forms between you and your baby as you both become increasingly involved in getting to know one another as unique individuals.

Unfortunately, however, many women soon become totally drained mentally, low in energy and sometimes even physically unwell, and find the responsibility of caring for a new baby overwhelming.

Using special aromatherapy treatments will encourage your rapid recovery following childbirth, helping combat fatigue, correct hormone imbalance, reduce discomfort, and enhance healing. Used in aromatic baths, compresses, massage, and topical treatments, essential oils will ensure that both you and your baby thoroughly enjoy this very special time. Remember that if you are feeling tense and anxious you will probably evoke the same response in your baby who will be irritable and difficult to settle. But equally, if you are calm and relaxed, the more soothing an effect you will have.

It is important for your recovery that you receive a nutritious diet and adequate amounts of rest and exercise. A daily short brisk walk is refreshing and can be enjoyed a few days after the birth. Why not take your baby along with you? Fresh air will help prevent infection developing, as well as ensuring settled sleep for you both.

There is always great excitement at the arrival of a new baby as friends and relatives visit. But entertaining a constant stream of guests throughout the day can be exhausting. It is therefore important that you limit visitors to sensible times that suit you. Do arrange for plenty of help with general household tasks as your partner may need as much support as you through the first few days, as all your time will be taken caring for your baby.

Make sure that you set aside some time for yourself each day. One good way is by relaxing in a warm aromatic bath. Add your favourite essential oils. Rose and Jasmine are not only two of nature's more luxurious essential oils but they do help restore your hormone balance, helping banish those 'baby blues'. Fluctuations in mood are experienced by most women, with emotions ranging from immense pride in the achievement of giving birth, to tears and feelings of anxiety that they may be unable to live up to the expectations and responsibilities of caring for a new baby.

If possible try to receive a regular aromatherapy massage from yourself, partner or aromatherapist, for massage will help reduce muscle tension and increase your vitality, making you feel better able to cope with those extra demands from your baby on your time and energy.

It is important always to recognize that you are not expected to work through your recovery without support. Make use of offers of help from friends and relatives, from doing your washing-up, to shopping or just watching your baby for a few hours while you rest. There are also many support groups available (see *Useful Addresses*) should you require specialist advice or the chance simply to share your concerns, and your midwife will also continue to visit regularly.

BREAST FEEDING

Many of the potential problems associated with breast feeding can be successfully treated with aromatherapy. Cracked nipples, insufficient milk, and too much milk leading to breast engorgement are among the most common complaints I have come across.

When breast feeding you can help prevent many problems developing by taking adequate amounts of rest, eating a nourishing diet, and drinking lots of mineral or filtered water to maintain your general health and fitness. Avoid alcohol and cigarettes as these harmful products pass easily into your breast milk, and you should also try to reduce the amount of coffee and tea you drink each day as these are stimulants with a high caffeine content which can make your baby restless and difficult to settle.

You should begin breast feeding as soon as possible after the birth. This stimulates the production of breast milk, as well as helping your uterus return to its normal size. Always feed your baby on demand with no restriction on the length of each feed. You may also find that your baby may feed on either one or both of your breasts in order to be satisfied at the end of a feed.

In the first few months of breast feeding, do not be tempted to give your baby any other food or fluid as your breast milk will provide all your baby's requirements for growth and development.

Breast engorgement can only be effectively reduced by feeding your baby, as initially your breasts will produce more milk than your baby actually requires. Quite quickly, however, milk production will settle into a process of supply and demand, in that eventually your breasts will produce only enough milk to replace the amount that has been drawn off at the previous feed. If you do become affected by breast engorgement, which may develop in the first few days when you begin to breast feed, the heat and pain you may experience can be relieved by applying cold Peppermint compresses. Cover the compress with a waterproof material inside a good supporting brassière, replacing the compress as soon as it warms to body temperature.

Cracked nipples can be avoided by correctly fixing your baby to your breast during breast feeding. Do not wash your nipples after every feed as this quickly dries out your skin, but clean them daily, then leave your skin to air dry. If you do begin to suffer from cracked nipples it is important that you seek immediate advice from your midwife or breast feeding counsellor so that the condition does not worsen. Meanwhile apply Calendula over the broken skin. Calendula has excellent healing properties, and there are many good proprietary brands available if you do not wish to make your own.

Although breast feeding is a completely natural activity, it may take a little while for you and your baby to get into the swing of things. Your midwife is on hand to advise you if you are unsure, as are many other specialists who can be contacted if you experience difficulties at home (see *Useful Addresses*).

BREAST MASSAGE

Mastitis can develop when your breasts have not completely emptied of milk, or if a milk duct becomes blocked. This can happen at any time once breast feeding is established, but I am convinced that by regularly practising breast massage with essential oils you will greatly reduce the likelihood of mastitis or the more serious condition of a breast abscess developing.

After each breast-feeding session, sit comfortably and slowly examine each breast in turn for any lumps, red or swollen areas. These usually indicate sites within your breast that have become affected.

If any of these signs are present apply a small amount of massage oil over the whole area. Use a carrier oil with a few added drops of Peppermint if your skin feels hot to the touch, or Rosemary if the area feels slightly swollen. Using your thumbs or finger pads massage with smooth strokes, working from just behind the problem area towards your nipple. You may feel a little resistance at first, but you will notice some improvement after a few minutes when you can begin to use still gentle but deeper strokes.

Continue your massage until the whole area softens. Finish off by gently massaging around your whole breast. Always work from the outer edge of your breast towards your nipple, remembering not to miss out your underarm area.

If stubborn areas persist after several minutes of massage, you may find it easier to continue your massage while soaking in a warm bath, or during breast feeding. Alternatively, try a different feeding position, such as lying on your side, which will help the affected area drain by gravity.

Even if you feel that your breasts have completely emptied of milk after feeding, do try to massage them at least once each day to prevent these potential problems developing.

Always remove all traces of essential oils before the next

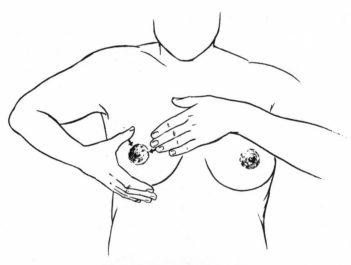

Fig. 19. Breast Massage

Apply a small amount of massage oil to your breast. Then, using your thumb or finger pads, massage with smooth strokes towards your nipple.

feed. This can be done quite easily using a mild soap and water solution.

A gentle breast massage should not feel unduly painful and should definitely not bruise your skin. Should your breasts become exceptionally painful or you develop a rise in body temperature you must seek further advice immediately as infection may be present. Even if mastitis does develop and you begin taking prescribed treatments, you can still continue breast feeding and should massage your breasts regularly to help the milk flow to relieve the congested areas. This will encourage healing and prevent your milk supply from drying up, so that you will be able to continue to feed properly throughout the period of infection, and afterwards.

HAEMORRHOIDS

Haemorrhoids, or piles as they are most commonly known, are varicose veins – damaged and swollen blood vessels, around the anus. If you are prone to haemorrhoids they may develop or worsen slightly during your pregnancy. It is important therefore to reduce extra strain by avoiding standing for long periods, avoiding exercises such as deep squatting, and making sure you do not suffer from constipation.

Haemorrhoids can become very swollen and painful following the birth of your baby, particularly if you have experienced a prolonged pushing stage. Therefore when labour begins it is always a good idea to inform your midwife if you were troubled with haemorrhoids during your pregnancy as this may influence your care during the birth of your baby. Your midwife may perhaps encourage you to give birth in an all-fours position, or may help support your haemorrhoids by applying pressure to them using a small pad of swabs or a clean folded sanitary towel.

If, after the birth of your baby, your haemorrhoids have

become enlarged, immediately apply ice packs wrapped in a soft clean material. These will help reduce the circulation and prevent further swelling. Then, as soon as possible, begin aromatherapy treatments.

Swelling and discomfort can be effectively reduced by applying Cypress oil. This powerful essential oil acts by helping to shrink and tone swollen blood vessels, and will help repair the damaged tissue. Add a few drops of Cypress oil to the tepid water of your bidet or sitz-bath, or use as a local wash after every visit to the toilet. Do not be tempted to apply Cypress oil in concentrated form as this may cause further tissue damage.

You can also use Cypress oil as a topical treatment diluted in a carrier oil. But when you apply this to your haemorrhoids use a mirror to help you, as this will enable you to avoid contact with any stitches or abrasions as healing may be impaired by the carrier oil.

You will probably find that your haemorrhoids are initially fairly slow to heal. However, with regular aromatherapy treatments you will feel an immediate improvement, followed by a gradual shrinkage, and eventual return to normal.

HEALING THE PERINEUM

Whether or not you require stitches following the birth of your baby you will probably experience a certain amount of discomfort in your perineum.

As soon as possible after birth apply ice packs to your perineum to help reduce tenderness and swelling. You can easily make your own ice packs by crushing ice cubes in a waterproof bag. Cover the ice pack with a piece of soft clean material, then apply very gently to your perineum.

In all but extreme cases, discontinue using ice packs after 24 hours, for unlike the treatment of haemorrhoids, the circulation to your perineum must be encouraged in order to stimulate healing. It is also important that you immediately begin to practise pelvic floor exercises several times each day. This will increase blood flow as well as strengthening the tissues that have become overstretched or damaged during the birth process. Natural healing does take place remarkably quickly, and aromatherapy treatments will help enhance this natural healing and reduce discomfort when it is difficult to find a comfortable position. Even though when you examine your perineum with a mirror there may be nothing to see externally, there may be some bruising of the deeper muscles under the skin.

Patchouli or Ti-Tree will help seal over the damaged tissue and encourage healing, helping reduce the formation of thick scar tissue. Add a few drops to the warm water of your bidet or sitz-bath, or use as a local wash after every visit to the toilet. Ti-Tree combines well with Lavender which will help protect you from infections developing and promote natural healing. Remember to cover your perineum with a clean sanitary towel after each treatment to keep the area clean and dry.

If a bidet is unavailable and bathing is difficult, add these essential oils to a container of warm water (an empty mineral water bottle can be kept specially for this purpose). You will find this method particularly useful if you are confined to bed, or using a urinary catheter (a fine latex tube used to drain the bladder). Simply sit over the toilet or on a bedpan and pour the solution over your vulva after washing, or use as a final rinse following vulval swabbing. Then dry the area well and cover with a clean sanitary towel.

After the birth of your baby, you may find that sitting down is uncomfortable to say the least! This can make life rather difficult especially when you are trying to establish breast feeding. In this case, try lying on your side until such time as you feel more comfortable sitting upright. Do not be tempted to use air or foam rings to support you. These have now been found to reduce the circulation to the perineum and to interfere with the healing processes as they tend to cause excess pressure on the sore areas.

12

YOU AND
YOUR BABY

Most women have their own special ideas of motherhood before their baby is born, with mental pictures of baby sleeping peacefully in the newly decorated nursery, while Mum gets on with her everyday life as before the birth.

Unfortunately, this picture is usually far from the truth. Most women wonder what they did to fill their days before their baby was born, finding that every waking moment is taken up with attending to the demands of her new baby, leaving her with little time to herself.

Of course, this period of adjustment lasts for a relatively short time, until you have recovered from the birth and you slowly become organized and tuned into recognizing your baby's needs. But the normal intense feelings of love that come with having a baby may also bring anger and frustration at times as you realize that your baby is totally dependent on you and you feel that you have lost all independence. These feelings are normal, but it is important that you use these emotions constructively. Make sure you are able to cope physically by arranging help from your partner, family and friends, and ensure that you have time for yourself.

If you have had no previous experience of caring for a small baby it would perhaps be a good idea if you could arrange for yourself and, if possible, your partner to visit a couple who have had a baby recently and who have passed successfully through this early stage. These visits can usually be arranged through your antenatal classes or birth group. During these visits you can experience handling and touching a small baby and obtain practical advice on coping with the early weeks of parenthood and, perhaps most importantly, discover that the feelings that you will experience are not unique.

Many women who are expecting subsequent babies often worry about the effects that a new addition to the family may cause, especially the response of older children. Unfortunately there is no ideal way of introducing older children to the new baby, or predicting how they will react, but a good start is to involve your children in your pregnancy and the development of the baby. Most children enjoy talking to their baby, feeling the baby kick against their mother's belly, and listening to the heart beat.

At the birth, try to minimize the length of separation from your family. A home birth may be ideal, or arrange for a shorter stay in hospital. As soon as possible involve your children in helping and caring for their baby.

Your children will enjoy holding and playing with the new baby and may like to join in the body massage sessions during which you could include a special massage for your older children using very diluted essential oils such as Rose or Lavender: 1 drop per 10 mls of carrier oil can be used safely.

I feel it is vitally important that you ensure that your older children feel as loved as they did before the arrival of the new baby, and that they understand that they will in fact receive lots of extra love from the new addition to their family.

13

BABY MASSAGE

Most parents instinctively stroke their babies right from the moment of birth as an unspoken welcome and to soothe the first cry. Baby massage is, I believe, a natural progression from this first moment of contact, especially for babies who have experienced the effects of massage through their mothers during life within the womb.

Today many hospitals, including the Neonatal Intensive Care Department within the maternity unit in which I am currently based, encourage parents to massage their babies at least once each day, for recent research has indicated that baby massage is beneficial to health and development.

You can massage your baby at any time of day, but do not massage if your baby has just had a feed.

Use a plain carrier oil. This is non-toxic, easily absorbed, and rich in nutrients that will help keep your baby's skin soft and supple. Add a little Wheatgerm oil if the skin is dry, but do not add essential oils as these are unsuitable for small babies.

Before you begin, wash your hands and remove any jewellery. Undress your baby, then lie your him or her on a soft clean towel, either on your lap or on the floor. Make sure that you keep your baby warm throughout the massage as babies lose body heat very quickly.

Pour a little massage oil into the palm of your hand, then rub your hands together to warm and evenly distribute the oil.

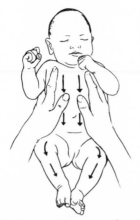

Fig. 20. Body Massage for Babies

Apply a little massage oil with long strokes down the whole length of the body.

Start with the head. Gently stroke the crown of the head, then with your fingertips smooth from the crown down the sides of the face (avoiding the delicate eye area).

Next, apply a little massage oil with long strokes down the whole length of the body (Figure 20). While massaging remember to maintain eye contact, play, talk or sing to your baby. This is reassuring for your baby as you discover which movements he or she enjoys. Repeat their favourite strokes 3 or 4 times.

Gently massage the belly with your fingertips using light circular clockwise strokes around the navel.

Massage each arm in turn. Circle the limbs with your hand and work hand over hand down towards the fingers. Then hold your baby's wrist, and massage the back of the hand and palm. Uncurl the fist and gently stroke and rotate each finger.

Move on to the legs. Work on each leg in turn, stroking with the flat of your hands down the leg towards the foot. Then, holding the feet at the ankles, massage over the whole surface of the foot with the pads of your thumbs (Figure 21). Gently stroke and rotate each toe in turn.

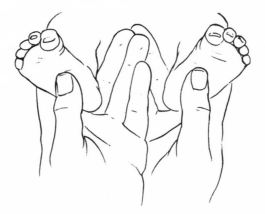

Fig. 21. Foot Massage for Babies

Holding the feet at the ankles, massage the whole surface of the foot using the pads of your thumbs.

Now turn your baby over to massage the back of the body. Apply a little more oil, again using long strokes down the whole length of the body. Stroke across the shoulders from the centre out, then down the length of the back using the palms of alternate hands on either side of the spine. Then gently massage over and around each buttock.

Finish off by repeating the long strokes down the whole length of the body several times, your hands gradually applying a softer, lighter pressure.

When you have completed your massage, cover your baby with a warm, soft, clean blanket or towel. By this stage your baby will be quite content to lie comfortably, or may even be sleepy. In either case allow your baby to rest for as long as they want.

You do not have to give a full massage each time. You may perhaps prefer to concentrate on areas that you feel will be particularly beneficial, such as the belly to relieve digestive upsets, or areas that you can reach easily, such as the face, hands or feet. But you will find that a daily full body massage will help soothe, quieten and reduce irritability as well as helping create a very special bond between you and your baby.

APPENDIX 1

VISITING YOUR AROMATHERAPIST: HOW TO FIND ONE AND WHAT TO EXPECT

Although this book is, I hope, a comprehensive guide to using aromatherapy during pregnancy and childbirth, the processes of selecting and blending essential oils do require a high level of skill and expertise. Therefore if you are considering using essential oils regularly, it is important that you first consult a fully trained aromatherapist.

You do not have to be ill to receive treatment, for aromatherapy is a preventative as well as a curative therapy. Most of us lead busy lives and we could all benefit from having a more relaxed mind and body. Having regular aromatherapy treatments is a good way of giving ourselves some time to unwind.

The best way of finding an aromatherapist is through personal recommendation from friends or relatives who have experienced treatments themselves. Alternatively, there are a number of professional organizations (see *Useful Addresses*) who will supply details of aromatherapists in your area. It may also be possible to obtain such information from your local supplier of essential oils.

Before you book your first appointment do check that your aromatherapist is suitably qualified from an approved school of training, and has practice insurance. This ensures that you receive only professional care and advice.

When you make an appointment you may be asked briefly to describe any problems that you feel need treatment. This gives the therapist the opportunity to make sure that aromatherapy is appropriate for you, and that you would not perhaps benefit from another type of complementary therapy, or a consultation with your general practitioner.

If you are seeing your general practitioner for a specific problem or have been prescribed medication, do tell your doctor that you are visiting an aromatherapist. You should also follow this rule if you begin to visit any other complementary therapist, such as an acupuncturist, homoeopath, or medical herbalist, as this can affect your treatments.

When deciding which therapist to visit do avoid those so-called 'aromatherapy' treatments that you may see advertised in beauty salons or hairdressers, as most use ready-mixed body preparations and massage blends rather than individually prescribed treatments based on a holistic diagnosis which assesses you as a whole person.

The first visit to an aromatherapist is usually the lengthiest, with appointments lasting between $1^{1}/_{2}$ and 2 hours. Subsequent sessions are usually about 1 hour in length, but can vary according to your therapist and the type of treatment you require.

Your aromatherapist will need to know about any medicines you have been prescribed or are currently taking. You will also be asked about your general health, diet, exercise and sleep pattern.

Having gathered all this information your aromatherapist will give you the opportunity to discuss any other problems that you feel are significant. All aspects of your life style, physical, mental and spiritual, are important for they all add up to a picture of your condition, and the underlying cause of any problems that you may be experiencing.

This consultation period is usually followed by a treatment session which, if appropriate, is usually a form of massage using a blend of essential oils carefully selected to meet your needs.

For a full body massage you will be asked to undress and lie on the massage couch covered with a large towel or blanket, while your aromatherapist prepares the massage oil. Throughout your massage you will be covered with towels and only the part of your body being massaged will be exposed. If, however, you find the idea of taking all your clothes off distressing, do inform your aromatherapist first who will then be able to work on those parts of your body which they believe will be the most effective – e.g. your head, neck and shoulders, back, hands or feet.

It is a good idea to wear clothes that can be easily removed and that will not be ruined by the massage oil. Jewellery and make-up should also be removed and, as most aromatherapists include a head massage, it is better to visit your hairdresser after your aromatherapist.

After your massage, your aromatherapist will probably leave the room giving you some time to relax quietly. When you feel ready to move, take several deep breaths in and out, stretch, turn on to your side, then sit up slowly before getting off the couch to get dressed.

Before you leave you may be asked if you wish to make another appointment. Do not feel under any obligation to book immediately, but if you are suffering from an acute condition you may wish to arrange several sessions in advance. Otherwise most women make appointments weekly, fortnightly, or monthly depending on time and finances.

Costs for consultation and treatment range from £10 to £25. Most aromatherapists are open to negotiation if you have a low income or you feel the need of an intensive course of treatment sessions. Many aromatherapists offer special discounts for treatments during pregnancy and childbirth, and often include baby massage sessions.

APPENDIX 2

HINTS ON SELECTING AND
BUYING ESSENTIAL OILS

Unfortunately there are no hard and fast rules when it comes to selecting and buying essential oils. Expense is no indication of quality, neither does buying a cheaper oil mean that you have found a bargain.

When inspecting the many brands available, you may discover some essential oils labelled as being organic. This indicates that the plant has been grown without the use of chemicals. Unfortunately there is no way of checking this fact, and such labelling could be used by unscrupulous suppliers as a way of raising prices. So beware!

Other suppliers may have a uniform price for their essential oils. This means that you will be paying a very high price for an essential oil that is less expensive to produce, or that the more expensive essential oils have been adulterated in some way to make them go further.

Do not buy essential oils that have already been blended or diluted in carrier oils as this will make it impossible for you to estimate the concentration and how much you will need to use in your own aromatic preparations.

Make sure that you only buy essential oils that are supplied in dark glass bottles as these protect their contents from deterioration during storage. Also check that they have droppers inserted for measuring the essential oils, and that the contents are suitably packaged to prevent contamination from strong-smelling odours or other shoppers eager to sample the essential oils before they buy them.

If you are still unsure about buying or selecting essential oils, ask the advice of your aromatherapist. If they are unable personally to provide you with the essential oils that you require, they will certainly be able to suggest a reliable supplier in your area. It is important that you obtain pure plant essences, as only these will give the desired healing effect.

CONCLUSION

I am a professionally qualified midwife and as such am the first to recognize the value of modern medicine and science in obstetric practice. I do, however, feel that these advances are sometimes abused and occasionally used as a matter of routine, when perhaps the more subtle natural therapies such as aromatherapy could be as effective. I therefore feel it is important during pregnancy and childbirth that you exercise your right to participate in your own care so that, apart from in an absolute emergency, you have the right to discuss any proposed treatments and, if appropriate, decide on the course of action you feel most comfortable with.

As an aromatherapist, I am encouraged that in addition to the many midwives who are practising aromatherapy, and the fact that baby massage is promoted as a form of care for premature or very ill babies and children, the use of aromatherapy is already established in many diverse areas of care. In units specializing in the treatment of serious illness, essential oils, massage and relaxation are respected as valuable forms of therapy. Aromatherapy is also being applied daily in the care of deeply unconscious patients who respond favourably to the stimulus of massage and the aroma of essential oils. And aromatherapy is also being slowly introduced into other areas such as care of the elderly and of patients affected by psychiatric disorders.

Aromatherapy is also slowly advancing into the workplace, as essential oils are frequently used in vaporizers to reduce the effects of environmental pollutants. Even massage sessions are provided by some progressive managers who recognize that aromatherapy is also a preventative therapy which will help reduce the loss of manpower through stress-related illness.

But having said all this, the future of aromatherapy remains uncertain, for within the next few years new laws are to be proposed to enforce stricter controls over the many practitioners of complementary therapies. In many ways these new laws will be a good thing in that they will ensure that all practising aromatherapists are professionally qualified, and will also guarantee the purity of all essential oils on sale. However, they may also make aromatherapy less accessible by allowing only those people who are also medically qualified to practise it, and it may become difficult for the general public to obtain essential oils and related products. Many believe that this type of law will be difficult to enforce, but a national body known as the Natural Medicines Society has been organized to promote the availability of all natural medicines (including aromatherapy) and welcomes the support of both practitioners and the general public (see *Useful Addresses*).

I do hope you will enjoy using aromatherapy for pregnancy and childbirth, and that afterwards, like me, you will become committed to the promotion and use of essential oils, and will continue to use aromatherapy personally and around your home for the benefit of your family and friends. In this way you will be helping to promote aromatherapy as well as making a positive contribution to health by using essential oils to reduce the stresses and strains of everyday life.

FURTHER READING

Books you may find interesting, giving further information on aromatherapy and related subjects, massage techniques, and pregnancy and childbirth:

Patricia Davis, *Aromatherapy An A-Z*, C. W. Daniel, 1988.

Julia Lawless, *The Encyclopaedia of Essential Oils*, Element, 1992.

Clare Maxwell-Hudson, *The Complete Book of Massage*, Dorling Kindersley, 1988.

Janet Balaskas and Yehudi Gordon, *The Encyclopaedia of Pregnancy and Birth*, Macdonald & Co., 1987.

USEFUL ADDRESSES

United Kingdom

Foresight
Association for the Promotion of
Preconceptual Care
28 The Paddock
Godalming, Surrey GU7 1XD
Tel: 01483 427839
Fax: 01483 427668

The Institute for
Complementary Medicine
PO Box 194
London SE16 1QZ
Tel: 0171 2375165
Fax: 0171 237 5175
*The Institute will supply details of
other complementary therapies.*

Active Birth Centre
Active Birth and Water Birth
25 Bickerton Road
London N19 5JT
Tel: 0171 561 9006
Fax: 0171 561 9007

The Natural Medicines Society
13a Market Place
Heanor
Derbyshire DE75 7AA
Tel: 01773 710002
Fax:01773 533855
This is a registered charity founded to

*protect and support the availability
and use of all plant medicines. It
welcomes support from both
professionals and the general public.*

National Childbirth Trust
Alexandra House
Oldham Terrace
London W3 6NH
Tel: 0181 992 8637

*The following will supply details of
accredited training schools and lists of
qualified aromatherapists:*
The International Society of
Professional Aromatherapists
82 Ashby Road
Hinckley
Leicestershire LE10 1SN
Tel: 01455 637987
Fax: 01455 890956

The International Federation of
Aromatherapists
Stamford House
2/4 Chiswick High Road
London W4 1TH
Tel: 0181 742 2605

Aromatherapy Organisations
Council
3 Latymer Close
Braybrooke
Market Harborough
Leicester
LE16 8LN
Tel: 01858 434242

Suppliers of essential oils and associated products:
The Fragrant Earth Co
PO Box 182
Taunton
Somerset TA1 3YR
Tel: 01823 335734
Fax: 01823 322566

Hermitage Oils
East Morton
Keighley
West Yorkshire BD20 5UQ
Tel: 01274 565957

Products:
Dept 2, Verde
15 Flask Walk
Hampstead
London NW3
Tel: 0870 603 9186

Australia

Action Pregnancy Problem Centre
228 Clarendon Street STE 5
East Melbourne
Victoria 3002
Australia
Tel: 613 9419 7622

Australian Natural Therapists
Association
PO Box 308
Melrose Park 5039
South Australia
Tel: 618 297 9533
Fax: 618 297 0003

International Federation of
Aromatherapists
PO Box 400
Balwyn Victoria 3103
Australia
IFA National Information Line:
190 224 0125

Childbirth Education Association
of Australia (NSW) Limited
Suite 11/127 Forest Road
Hurstville 2220
PO Box 413 Hurstville 2220
Australia
Tel: (02) 580 0399
Fax: (02) 580 9986

The Childbirth Education
Association (Brisbane) INC
PO Box 208
Chermside 4032
Australia
Tel: (07) 3359 9724

USA

The American Alliance of
Aromatherapy
PO Box 750428
Petaluma
CA 94975
Tel: 707 778 6762

The American Alliance of
Aromatherapy
PO Box 309
Depoe Bay
Oregon 97341
USA
Tel: (800) 809 9850
Fax: (800) 809 9808

Australia

Australian Natural Therapists
Association
PO Box 308
Melrose Park 5039
South Australia
Tel: 618 297 9533

Australian Traditional Medicine
Society Limited
PO Box 1027
Meadow Bank
NSW 2114

Childbirth Education Association
of Australia Limited
Suite 11
127 Forest Road
Hurstville 2220
NSW
Tel: 02 580 0399

The Childbirth Education
Association Inc
PO Box 208
Chermside 4032
Brisbane
Tel: 07 3359 9724

Canada

Canadian Holistic Medical
Association
700 Bay Street
PO Box 101
Suite 604
Toronto
Ontario M5G 1Z6

Nature Trading Limited
Box 263
1857 West 4th Avenue
Vancouver
V63 1M4

Ireland

Wholefoods Wholesale
Unit 2D
Kylemore Industrial Estate
Dublin 10

Soap Opera Limited
Unit 3
Enterprise Centre
Stafford Street
Nenagh
Co Tipperary

*Some of the addresses are professional
organizations, some give their
services free of charge. Please
remember to enclose a stamped
addressed envelope with your initial
enquiry.*

INDEX